Policy Options in
Long-Term Care

Edited by
Judith Meltzer,
Frank Farrow, &
Harold Richman

Policy Options in Long-Term Care

The University of Chicago Press
Chicago and London

The University of Chicago Press, Chicago 60637
The University of Chicago Press, Ltd., London

Library of Congress Cataloging in Publication Data
Main entry under title:

Policy options in long-term care.

   Papers from a national Symposium on Long-Term-
Care Policy Options held in Williamsburg, Va., in
June 1980.
   Bibliography: p.
   Includes index.
   1. Long-term care of the sick—Government policy
—United States—Congresses.   2. Long-term care of
the sick—United States—Congresses.   I. Meltzer,
Judith.   II. Farrow, Frank.   III. Richman, Harold,
1937–   IV. Symposium on Long-Term-Care Policy
Options (1980: Williamsburg, Va.)
RA644.6.P64   362.1'6'0973   81-10445
ISBN 0-226-51973-2 (cloth)   AACR2
ISBN 0-226-51974-0 (pbk.)

Contents

7   **Cost Estimation and Long-Term-Care Policy**
Problems in Forecasting the Undefined   209
Jay Greenberg and William Pollak

Acknowledgments

We are especially indebted to Tom Joe, Carol Estes, and Phil Lee for their early work in initiating this project and for their continued guidance throughout.

We wish to thank the Administration on Aging of the U.S. Department of Health and Human Services for their financial support of this work. The staff there who assisted us were Commissioner Robert Benedict, Byron Gold, Harry Posman, and Richard Hoke.

We owe special thanks to the members of the Project Steering Committee who helped define the areas of study and provided criticism, suggestions, and guidance: Charles Burger, Lewis Butler, Carol Estes, Jay Greenberg, Tom Joe, Phil Lee, Bentley Lipscomb, Laurence Lynn, George Moran, Bernice Neugarten, Robert Patricelli, Henry Russe, Brahna Traeger, and Stanley Wallack. Bernice Neugarten was particularly helpful in a number of ways.

We are also grateful to our colleagues Don Simpson and Cheryl Rogers, to Kathy Sheehan, who managed the project in its early stages, and to Patricia Young and Adele Barden, who did much of the typing.

Preface

One of the most pressing policy problems facing the nation in the next decade is developing ways to meet the needs of persons with chronic functional impairments. The long-term-care problem, as it has come to be called, has become a major domestic priority. It is an area in which there has been almost as much difficulty in framing the issues as in proposing solutions. Recognition of the long-term-care problem and a sense of urgency about responding to it have been building, not only because of the growing numbers of people seemingly at risk but because of the continuing and sharp increase in public expenditures for institutional long-term care. Numerous constituencies (professionals, politicians, taxpayers, and persons in need of care) are recognizing that the ways in which long-term-care services are financed, organized, and made available are fraught with problems. Much of the frustration has focused on inadequacies in caring for those who suffer from chronic disabilities. Many of these persons are old, but the problem cannot be limited or defined by age. The problems of long-term care have become a symbol of America's traditional rejection of dependency and seeming callousness to the problems that accompany chronic illness and disability.

Concern about the lack of productive debate on long-term care provided the impetus for the national Symposium on Long-Term-Care Policy Options held in Williamsburg, Virginia, in June, 1980, and supported by the Administration on Aging of the U.S. Department of Health and Human Services.

This book has grown out of the symposium's focus on major unresolved long-term-care policy issues that have received inadequate attention in the planning and political process. The issues include:

1. Developing an awareness and beginning consensus on the goals and objectives of long-term-care policy—for example, what is to be accomplished and what values should be maximized by future policy directions?

2. Determining the nature and extent of public responsibility for meeting the long-term-care needs of the population. What should be the amount, scope, and direction of public support compared with the responsibilities and preferences of individuals, families, and private philanthropy?

3. Providing guidance on the practical and political choices governing the allocation of scarce public resources, including who should be served, to what extent, and how.

4. The difficult job of designing a system or systems to deliver the necessary services to people.

In examining these issues, we have deliberately tried to move the public debate beyond the frustrating morass of problem identification and conflicting ad hoc solutions. The entire effort was guided by a national steering committee composed of persons with wide experience in the government, academia, and the private sector. The steering committee was responsible for framing the issues requiring further analysis, and it commissioned and assisted in the development of the policy papers included in this volume. The papers were subsequently reviewed by the steering committee and an additional group of national experts who participated in the two-day working symposium. The introductory paper was written after the other six. Taken together, the seven papers critically examine the pressing questions in the long-term-care policy debate. In doing so, they bring together much of what is now known in this field. The papers provide thoughtful insight on the nature of the problems, the need for change, and possible directions for reform. Although the papers benefited from the insights of those involved in the symposium process, they represent the views of the authors.

It seems certain that during the next several years the nation will, both by choice and by necessity, attempt to develop policies and programs to meet the needs of persons who suffer from chronic functional impairments. It is our hope that this work will be a positive contribution to this policy development.

1

Introduction
The Framework and
Directions for Change

Frank Farrow, Tom Joe,
Judith Meltzer, and
Harold Richman

Introduction

I am an 84 year old woman, and the only crime I have committed is that I have an illness that is called chronic. I have severe arthritis and about five years ago I broke my hip. While I was recuperating in the hospital, I realized that I would need extra help at home. But there was no one. My son died 35 years ago; my husband, 25 years ago . . . so I wound up at a convalescent hospital.

I have been keeping in touch with the world through the newspaper, my one great luxury. For the last few years I have been reading about changes in Medicare regulations. All I can see from these improvements is that nurses spend more time writing. For, after all, how do you regulate caring? . . . There are a few caring people who work here, but there are so many of us who are needy for that kind of honest attention.

In the five years I have been here, I have had no choice—no choice of when I want to eat or what I want to eat. . . . How can I begin to tell you that growing old in America is for me an unbelievable, lonely nightmare? . . . Right now, I pray that I may die in my sleep and get this nightmare of what someone has called life over with, if it means living in this prison day after day.

Anonymous, *Los Angeles Times,* September 23, 1979

The letter reprinted above dramatically highlights problems associated with caring for the chronically ill and dependent. The example is of an older person, but similar problems exist for people across the age spectrum. The need to expand the available choices for this woman and countless others is the primary motivation for change in current programs and policies.

Examining the issues in the long-term-care policy debate is complicated by the imprecision of the phrase long-term care itself. To some, it is synonymous with nursing homes; to others, with the elderly and the process of growing old in America. We propose the following definition:

1

Long-term care represents a range of services that address the health, social, and personal care needs of individuals who, for one reason or another, have never developed or have lost some capacity for self care. Services may be continuous or intermittent, but it is generally presumed that they will be delivered for the "long term," that is, indefinitely to individuals who have a demonstrated need, usually measured by some index of functional incapacity.[1]

There are several components of this definition which merit attention. First, long-term care is related to demonstrated individual need, which is presumably measured by some level of functional limitation rather than by assumed membership in an at-risk category (i.e., those who are 65 or older or 75 or older). As Bernice Neugarten has written:

While it is true that, overall, the frequency of illness and disability increases with age in the latter part of life, the association between age and physical capacity is far from perfect and it sets very wide limits within which individual variation is the important reality. This being the case, it does not help much in predicting a person's health, or marital status, or economic status, or life satisfaction, to know only that the person is 60 rather than 50, or 70 rather than 60. This is a finding that has emerged over and over as research accumulates and it is this generalization that gerontologists have in mind when reporting that in the second half of life age is a poor predictor of physical or intellectual or social performance. In this sense, age is becoming a less relevant characteristic than it was in earlier periods of our history.[2]

There are limitations in our ability to measure individual need based on functional limitations or any other criterion, but we believe there is no inherent justification (other than strategic considerations for legislation or administrative change) for tying the definition of long-term care to an arbitrary criterion like age or for using an age cutoff. Long-term-care policies must be concerned not only about the needs of the elderly, but also with the problems of children and younger adults with chronic functional impairments.[3]

Second, the definition acknowledges that needs vary between individuals and change over time, requiring diverse, flexible, and individualized responses. Long-term care is a term which incorporates a wide variety of dependency needs which differ for individuals in a given social situation. There is no neat translation from need to response, and, even as plans are established, they must be flexible and respond to changes in an individual's condition or in the familial and community context of the service provision. As James Callahan states, a system of long-term care should be

capable of achieving at least one of the following goals for each person
served based on his/her individual situation:
1. Maximum functional independence at all times, even if there are limitations in activity or deterioration of function.
2. Rehabilitation, in order to restore some previous level of functioning
   which can be sustained.
3. Humane care for persons functionally and permanently dependent.
4. Utilization of the least restrictive environment for care.
5. Death with dignity.[4]

   Third, the definition incorporates income maintenance, health, housing,
personal care, and social services. All of them are necessary components
of long-term-care services, and their interrelationship and/or lack of it is
often a major source of complexity and problems in the provision of care.
An adequate income is the essential base, a fact often overlooked in
discussions of long-term-care service provision. While most chronically
impaired persons have some income through Social Security (old age and
disability payments), Supplemental Security Income (SSI), and private
pensions, the lack of an adequate income is a severe problem for many,
especially in these times of rapid inflation. Debate about the adequacy of
income support for long-term-care populations is important particularly in
light of the fact that even with Social Security, SSI, and private pensions,
the rate of poverty for older and disabled persons is disproportionately
high and increases with advancing age.[5] Housing as a component of
long-term-care services has also received far too little attention, particularly the development of congregate or group living arrangements which
encourage support networks of family and friends and facilitates access to
other needed services. Health care, including primary and acute care and
continuing care for the management of chronic illness, is another essential
component. The health care aspects of long-term care predominate in
current financing and delivery. But even with respect to health care there
has been underattention to continuing management of chronic illness and
overemphasis on acute services and care in institutional settings. The
provision of personal care and social services, particularly those that
would enable persons to continue to live in their own homes, is the
weakest aspect of current long-term-care service provision. The need to
develop social support resources and systems for financing and providing
personal care and social services (i.e., day care, homemaker, chore services, respite care, nutrition services, socialization, counseling) is a major
focus of our recommendations.

   Fourth, the definition implies a continuum of care, encompassing preventive care and acute care as well as continuous care over a long period
of time.

Finally, the definition does not prescribe either the auspices of the provider (i.e., public/private, formal/informal) or the locus of service provision (home, community, or institution). A flexible response to individual needs and preferences must incorporate many different kinds of providers (medical and nonmedical) and both community-based and institutional care.

Before any discussion of the context for policy change, it is important to underscore the damaging misconceptions that pervade the subject area. All too often, concern about meeting the needs of the dependent elderly and handicapped leads us to assume that all elderly and disabled need long-term care. Public policy must be concerned with the needs of the dependent, but be equally careful to avoid stereotypes that assume that overwhelming incapacities and frailties invariably accompany old age and disability. Those with chronic functional impairments, including disabled young adults and older persons who now require and will continue to require substantial supports in daily functioning, possess personal skills and strengths which must be recognized and enhanced, rather than supplanted with paternalistic public programs. This perspective has implicitly guided this paper and must, in our opinion, undergird long-term-care policy development.

II. The Context for Future Policy Development

Before we examine the major directions for future long-term-care policy, it is useful to review factors which will influence the nature, scope, and pace of change in this field.

Perhaps the most important factor is that the need for long-term care is growing and will continue to grow in both the short term and the more distant future. The long-term-care debate has focused on the needs of individuals over age 65. According to a staff report to the Federal Council on Aging Task Force on the Frail Elderly,[6] approximately 19.9 percent of individuals over age 75 can be classified as "frail elderly" and thus at risk of needing long-term care. Demographic projections of the future size and characteristics of the elderly population indicate that the proportion of older people in this age range will continue to grow, with the aged population as a whole doubling by the year 2035.[7] Thus, public officials are aware that the need for long-term-care services will grow accordingly.

In addition to the growing population of elderly persons with chronic conditions, adult disabled persons comprise a substantial portion of the population with long-term-care needs. Approximately 23 percent of the population over 18 years old have at least some limitations in their physical functioning.[8] Recently analyzed data indicate that the number of adult disabled under age 65 who have severe impairments is equal to the number of people over 65 with impairments.[9] Yet, only an estimated one-third of the five to ten million adults who may have needed long-term-care services in 1975 were receiving them.[10]

Much of the impetus for long-term care reform stems from the escalating cost of such care for federal and state governments. Long-term-care costs have skyrocketed since 1965 and continue to increase at an alarming pace. Over $11 billion in public and private funds were spent on long-term-care services in fiscal year 1975, representing a 200 percent increase from 1970.[11] Most of this increase was caused by institutional care costs (skilled nursing and intermediate care facilities), which have increased more rapidly and have proven more inflationary than other health care costs. Of total national expenditures for nursing home care in 1978 ($15.751 billion), Title XIX (Medicaid) was the primary source of public support, paying 46 percent of the costs of care, or $7.2 billion. This is an increase from $3.9 billion in 1974.[12] The pressure an increase of this magnitude puts on federal and state budgets is clear.

Thus there are two major aspects of the demand for change in long-term care: (1) expanded and improved care, particularly community-based care, and (2) control of costs. There is disagreement on the extent to which these two goals are compatible; in many cases, states as well as the federal government are attempting to pursue both goals simultaneously, with the tradeoffs between care and costs being unclear.

Despite the difficulties that have been encountered, change in long-term-care policy is already under way. The pressure for more responsive federal long-term-care policies and programs has been increasing for some time, and alterations in the major federal programs related to long-term care have been proposed or enacted. The 1978 changes in the Older Americans Act (OAA) regulations are an example. Although evidence suggests that they have not been fully implemented, the regulations target services to the elderly "with greatest economic, social need" and require a statewide long-term care ombudsman program.[13] Similarly, the recent home health report submitted to the Congress by the Department of Health and Human Services (HHS)[14] outlines systematic changes in Medicaid, Medicare, and Title XX regulations and legislation that would make home health care under these programs more equitable and accessible. The channeling initiative launched by HHS[15] in September 1980 represents a further effort to test methods for improved community-based long-term care, and the designs of the funded projects incorporate aspects of long-term-care service delivery clearly important to federal policy.

State governments on their own are changing long-term-care policies and priorities. Although the major funding for both institutional and noninstitutional long-term care is federal, most of this financing is through programs over which states have considerable policy and administrative control. Lacking effective federal direction in this field, states have attempted a variety of approaches either to expand community-based services, or to control the growth of institutional care, or both.

In short, the issue seems no longer to be if changes in long-term-care policy will occur, but how, under whose auspices, and at what pace. More importantly, the question is whether new policies affecting long-term care will be developed within a commonly defined framework for federal policy or on an ad hoc basis without benefit of coordination across programs, across agencies, and among levels of government. As will be clear, a premise of this paper and of the subsequent papers in this volume is that change in long-term care should be guided by overall federal policy direction, within which states are able to formulate and administer programs which can be adapted to state needs. The intergovernmental complexity of existing long-term-care programs cannot be disregarded as new policies are developed. Any viable federal policy must build on present federal, state, and local relationships, explicitly considering the role of states in setting priorities and developing implementation plans. To do otherwise is to ignore the fact that state and local agencies now control most of the financing streams for which redeployment is necessary if effective long-term-care delivery systems are to be built.

Although fiscal constraints must be recognized, they should not control federal and state policy decisions to the extent that long-run goals for long-term care are sacrificed. Present long-term-care financing is seriously flawed in part because it arose as a series of ad hoc solutions to a persistent and deepening set of problems. The failure to articulate a policy goal related to a continuum of long-term care and to work gradually toward that goal has led to the overly expensive and institutionally oriented system which we now face.

The lesson seems to be that present policy decisions should accommodate themselves to the realities of likely financing, at the same time building toward a more comprehensive system of care.

Clearly, the preceding assumption puts a premium on long-term-care strategies which redeploy existing resources more effectively, which create necessities for private investment, and which contain incentives for cost control. Even if new dollars are allocated to long-term care, the first necessary step is to gain better control over the large sums already directed to the care of impaired persons. A corollary of this principle is that the implementation of our major strategies for change will require programmatic and fiscal phasing-in over time.

Finally, the discussion of policy options in this paper and in the other papers of this volume is undertaken with a realization that information necessary for certain critical choices is currently lacking. In fact, the scarcity of empirical evidence on the likely costs or outcomes of expanded noninstitutional long-term care is often the reason cited for the lack of a coherent federal long-term-care policy and strategy, or for the inevitability of incremental change rather than bolder steps. In the discussion of future directions which follows, we are explicit where information should be obtained before certain choices are made. Information gaps can be addressed through research, demonstrations, and other techniques for obtaining new knowledge. Acknowledging such information gaps, we have attempted to narrow the range of options and suggest preferences, based on the information currently available. This reflects an assumption that sufficient knowledge does exist to proceed with improvements in both the financing and service delivery of long-term care. Basic policy choices must be made at the same time that more definitive information is being developed with regard to the needs for, demand for, and costs of long-term care. Research and demonstration efforts, however, must be more carefully designed to contribute to policy decisions.

It is within this context that long-term-care strategies must be designed, enacted, and implemented if care of chronically impaired people is to be improved substantially. This has not been a simple task in the past and promises to pose continued difficulties in the future. The context within which reform must be pursued is not the only barrier to change, however. There remains a core group of policy problems related to long-term care which must be analyzed and resolved if effective financing and delivery strategies are to emerge. We turn now to a discussion of those issues which serve as the necessary background for considering alternative policy directions. Each is discussed briefly in this paper, and at greater length in the papers which follow.

III. Policy Problems

There have been many analyses of the problems with the current system of long-term care.[16] The intent here is not to catalog all of the ills in the current provision of long-term care, but to emphasize those issues which have been given insufficient attention in the past, and which remain troublesome as new directions are sought.

The most important policy problem is a lack of consensus about the nature and extent of public responsibility for meeting long-term-care needs. This results in an inability to articulate a coherent set of goals and directions for future policy development. As stated by Elizabeth Kutza,

The decision to mount a national program for the provision of long-term care is a most serious one. It involves explicit acknowledgment of the role of the state regarding certain dependent groups, acceptance of a commitment that may be costly and far-reaching, and it comes at a time when our financial resources are contracting. The choices now facing us are difficult, influenced by legal imperatives, public attitudes, economic and political constraints. Yet choices must be made.[17]

The extent of public responsibility for long-term care cannot be thought of as an absolute. Current long-term-care services reflect the available financing mechanisms (i.e., Medicare, Medicaid, SSI, Title XX, OAA) more than they reflect conscious and deliberate decisions about what kinds of services ought to be made available to what people under what conditions. The extent of public responsibility for care depends on social values, patterns of family behavior, and the awareness of need as perceived by legislators, public officials, and other decision makers. As Robert and Rosalie Kane have suggested, public and private responsibilities exist in a

> state of regularly recalibrated equilibrium. Private initiative responds to public cues offered by funding sources and also to the need to provide uncovered services. Public responsibility for long-term care can, in part, be defined as filling in the voids not met by other systems, both formal and informal.[18]

Because public programs providing long-term care have not evolved from a unified policy direction, the resulting service system is at best inconsistent, incoherent, and fragmented and varies enormously from state to state and within states.

However, momentum is developing for changing the extent and nature of public responsibility for long-term care. Callahan has identified potential pressures for change, including the demographic shifts discussed earlier; an expanded pool of long-term-care professionals and provider interest groups; and new consciousness and political awareness among potential client groups and affected individuals.[19] These forces, combined with widespread concern about the increasing and seemingly uncontrollable costs of current patterns of care, may well provide the necessary impetus for the development of a more coherent federal policy.

A major concern in developing policy for the future is that *any expansion of public responsibility for long-term care not jeopardize existing familial and informal care arrangements.* All of the papers highlight the need to establish partnerships between families and formal services and to develop public policies which underpin informal supports and capacities. In discussing need for long-term services, Kutza cites the existence of social supports as a major variable influencing the utilization of formal services:

Increasingly, studies identify a community network as key in explaining differences in utilization of long-term-care services. . . . For the functionally limited adult, the main source of support is the spouse. The importance of the spouse is reflected in nursing home resident data that show three times as high a proportion of persons who have never been married and twice as high a proportion of widowed persons.[20]

This finding is supported by Lewis Butler and Paul Newacheck's data analysis which confirms other findings that social factors (particularly marital status and living arrangements) are highly significant in determining who is at risk of being institutionalized.[21]

Kutza goes on, however, to emphasize the fragility of informal caretaking arrangements, citing a New England study showing that there was a significant drop-off in families' ability and willingness to care for relatives after a second hospitalization.[22]

That study and other research[23] support the view that, when available, families and informal supports are critical but that there is wide disparity in their availability across the population and that such informal supports need to be assisted by formal care-giving arrangements. The danger, however, is that expanded public intervention may not support but supplant existing informal patterns of care.

There is a clear need to maintain informal care providers as part of the long-term-care system. Unfortunately, the rhetoric in support of informal care arrangements exceeds our knowledge of how to preserve this type of care. Several of the policy options discussed later in this paper are designed to maximize care from family and relatives by providing income subsidies for this care. Beyond financial support, however, few methods have been suggested to ensure that care by families is not replaced.

A third policy issue centers on the definition of need for long-term-care services and what criteria ought best be used in defining the nature and extent of the need. After a review of data, Kutza concludes:

> There remain serious questions about who needs care. Disability or functional limitation appears to be a necessary but not sufficient condition of risk for long-term care. Not all persons within high-risk categories (the very old, the disabled, the chronically mentally ill) are dependent upon others for care, and those who are dependent have needs that vary in intensity, duration, and scope.[24]

At issue in the policy debate is the relationship between need, however defined, and eligibility decisions. Several choices exist. Need can be based on (1) membership in an at-risk population group (i.e., the elderly, the disabled, the mentally handicapped); (2) membership in a population group defined by a combination of at-risk factors (i.e., poverty, age, social

isolation, taken together); (3) a diagnosis of functional limitations, irrespective of other factors; or (4) functional limitations, but with consideration of other resources available to the individual in determining the services to be made available.

There are problems with each of these options. We know, for example,
that increasing age, although associated with increased need for long-
term-care services, is not in itself an equitable service-rationing criterion.
As Butler and Newacheck show, there is no abrupt decline in health
status at 65 or any particular age.[25] For most persons, the decline is
gradual, becoming apparent in middle age and building steadily up
through the 85-plus group. Their analysis of the disability data leads them
to conclude that classifying persons by age and using such terms as the
"frail elderly" and "old old" are misleading and inappropriate to public
policy.

The presence of a functional limitation is perhaps a better measure of
need, but current tools for measuring functional abilities are primitive at
best. As Kutza states,

> The major shortcoming of functional assessment tools is that the level of
> functioning they measure is not readily translated into need for service.
> For example, a person may score poorly on mobility. A response to
> that problem can take various forms—a wheelchair, a walker, a cane,
> better shoes, podiatry services.[26]

The judgment of need is usually a professional decision based on widely
varying assumptions and standards and including an evaluation of service
options available to the disabled person. For policy planners, the issue is
further complicated by the unclear relationship between need for a service
and subsequent demand and utilization. Estimates of demand and utilization are essential if we are to be able to project realistically the costs of
any proposed programs. However, as Kutza notes, the level of demand
for services is a complex mixture of individual preference and the price of
services. In addition, family attitudes, social structures, and the
availability of informal support may be critical determinants of demand
for and utilization of long-term-care services. This alternative thus poses
problems of equity. If two individuals have equal need based on degree of
functional limitation, but one person has a spouse who provides care
while the other lives alone, should the public assessment of "need" reg-
ister only the solitary individual? Clearly, the issue of determining need is
entangled with the basic decisions on appropriate public responsibility for
care.

A related issue centers on *the difficulty of allocating scarce resources in the absence of any clear definitions of need or conceptually defensible eligibility criteria.* While most observers theoretically would support the notion that services be universally available to all those in need, it is equally true that it is unlikely that public resources will be able to support a universal entitlement program in the near future. This is especially important in light of the current spiraling inflation and public reaction in terms of limited governmental expenditures at the federal, state, and local levels.[27] The reality of fiscal constraint requires strategic consideration of rationing public resources by use of such devices as means tests, copayment mechanisms which would cut down utilization, or eligibility restrictions based on severity of need.

Each of these rationing devices has problems. For example, means tests usually raise concern about a dual system—a public welfare program for the poor with all of its presumed attendant stigma and frequent inadequacies, and a private system for those who can afford it. This may be less of an issue than assumed, considering the high prevalence of poverty among older and disabled people. In 1978, the median income for families headed by a person over 65 was 43.5 percent lower than the median income for all families. Fifty percent of all elderly have incomes of less than twice the poverty line; in 1978 this was $7,232 for an individual and $7,834 for a couple.[28] Perhaps a closer examination of the population at risk combined with an appreciation of the high cost of long-term-care services will force us to reconsider our negative assumptions about means tests. Rationing based on severity of need raises equally, if not more, troubling issues, such as the trade-off of preventive services for treatment beginning only after progressive deterioration. Many argue that intervention at the later point is too little, too late. Further, given the changing nature of individual conditions and needs, there are difficult practical problems with objectively setting and measuring disability levels appropriate for intervention.

The next two policy problems move us from a consideration of who should be served to questions of how and what kind of services should be provided. One of the most troublesome problems with our current care system is the *medicalization of long-term-care financing and services* and its resulting *overemphasis on institutional and acute care.* The problem of altering the balance of care from acute medical and institutional care is a serious one since all of the current financing and most of the professional incentives go in that direction. As Lee and Estes have written:

> Long-term care has been medicalized, because this was the only avenue open to support the development of needed services. In the process, however, long-term care has been accorded a low priority, be-

cause physicians and hospitals find it less prestigious and economically rewarding than acute care. Institutional care has been emphasized at the expense of community and home care services. Nursing homes have been required to perform multiple functions—custodial care, acute illness care, rehabilitation, chronic care, and terminal care—without the resources to perform these tasks. Alternative policies for income maintenance and housing have not been adequately considered, because the medical model has been so dominant and so costly.[29]

The medicalization of long-term care is especially troubling in view of our increased understanding of the kinds of problems presented by the long-term-care population. The Butler/Newacheck paper strongly argues against this acute care/medical bias, based on their findings that people become vulnerable to institutionalization not so much from a change in health status, as from a change in marital status and living arrangements. They conclude that

> considering those persons most at risk, the disabled living alone, the chances that added medical spending will reduce the risk of institutionalization seem slight. . . . In contrast, added dollars for housing, nutrition, and other services may assist the elderly in improving their lives.[30]

Within the medical care system, they emphasize the need for continuous management of chronic illness in community settings rather than the predominant provision of episodic, acute care in hospitals and other medical institutions. An additional troubling paradox is that even for those within highly medical settings like nursing homes, appropriate provision of primary medical care is often lacking.

The need to redress the medical care imbalance in existing programs relates to another theme of this paper that a *major shortcoming in long-term care is the absence of personal care services and other social supports which can assist the individual to remain in the community.* The existence of such community social support systems with links to the income maintenance system, housing, and adequate health care is a critical missing element of public policy. The difficulty of establishing the necessary community social supports and tying them to other ongoing systems of care is underscored in Callahan's discussion of the "intersystem" concept.[31]

In analyzing the characteristics of the current delivery system, Callahan notes that long-term-care services are now provided by many human service subsystems (health, housing, income maintenance, education, employment, personal social services). There are ill-defined boundaries and links between these system which cause problems for the long-term-care client. Further, the long-term-care client in most of these cases is marginal to the service providers upon which he or she depends and thus has little priority in claiming resources.[32] Callahan further concludes that the subsystem which may be most important to the long-term-care client, the personal social service system, is poorly organized and barely exists as a system. The implication is that even if we can address adequately the issues posed by intersystem boundaries and marginality, we still will need to develop resources in the area of personal care and social supports.

An additional policy problem is the *scant attention given to appropriate housing as a critical component of long-term care.* One reason that institutional care has been the dominant form of long-term care is that it provides services within a housing arrangement. Particularly for impaired people living alone, lack of suitable housing is a major barrier to community-based living. Their housing may be too costly or too difficult to maintain, and may impose barriers to activities of daily living or reinforce isolation.

Yet the issue of housing has not been a major part of the long-term-care debate. To some extent, this inattention to housing seems to reflect a fear that any long-term-care strategy which calls for new forms of housing or alternative living arrangements will prove prohibitively expensive. Also, there is little experience with innovative housing arrangements for impaired people. The debate has focused on institutional versus home care, with almost no attention given to other types of supported living or congregate housing.

The categorical provision of current services and Callahan's intersystem concept highlight another issue which deserves special attention, that is, *how to achieve coordination of and access to the multiple human services needed by many long-term-care clients.* In current professional jargon, this has become tied to the concepts of case management and channeling. (We will discuss channeling agencies in more detail below.) As Callahan has noted,

> Because the disabled person partakes of these different subsystems, a need for case coordination . . . is presumed. . . . While this is a reasonable assumption with many case examples to support it, the number of persons requiring case coordination is not known, nor are the nature and extent of required linkages among the subsystems.[33]

We have tended to assume a widespread need for case management in this area with very few data to support such an assumption. Case management has become so much taken for granted that it has been elevated to an independent professional service (often substituting for other needed services). It is highly probable that some portion of the long-term-care population will require active case management. We should be careful, however, not to build a long-term-care system around it without better understanding the needs of the population, and the manpower and cost implications of greatly expanded mechanisms of coordination and client management.

A final problem which constrains the development of national long-term-care policy is the *wide variation in current patterns of state and local financing and availability of services.* This variation grows out of the categorical federal programs which give states and localities considerable decision-making latitude about program priorities, service definitions, and recipient eligibility. The benefits made available under categorical federal-state programs are heavily influenced by the state's willingness and ability to share in the costs of the services,[34] as well as by competing pressures brought to bear on state and local officials by taxpayers, service providers, and current and potential beneficiaries.

The major federal programs supporting long-term-care services fall within the discretion of state policies and services (i.e., Medicaid, Title XX, SSI, OAA). According to the Congressional Budget Office (CBO), Medicaid expenditures accounted for 77 percent of government-financed long-term care in 1977. Within broad federal guidelines, however, states are free to define the eligibility, scope, amount, and duration of covered services. The Medicaid home health care benefit is a perfect example. Although a required service, home health benefits constitute about .1 percent to .5 percent of total Medicaid expenditures in most states. Even within this small total expenditure, there is a critical imbalance among the states. New York State alone accounted for 63 percent of all home health recipients served in 1976 and 81 percent of all federal home health payments in FY 1977.[35] Under the Title XX program, states can provide a wide range of in-home services. Again, there is considerable state variation; California, for example, spent about 10 to 15 percent of its Title XX funds on such services. Finally, under the federal SSI program, states are free to supplement the federal benefit for state-defined categories of protective living arrangements. Thirty-four states provides such supplementation with benefits for individuals varying widely among states and within states depending on the nature and definition of the congregate care facility.

The resolution of the policy problems discussed here in part depends on one's overall view of the appropriate direction for change. Different policy directions imply different solutions to these issues. Before making our recommendations, we thus turn to a consideration of alternative directions.

IV. Alternatives for Change

The four alternatives presented here offer significantly different choices and incorporate significantly different perspectives about the nature and extent of federal responsibilities for long-term care. The alternatives are not discrete, mutually exclusive options; combinations of these directions are possible and desirable, and in the real world it is likely that combinations or some mixture of two or more of these alternatives may even be inevitable.

The alternatives differ primarily in (1) the federal, state, and local roles considered appropriate in the development of long-term-care financing and resources; (2) the financing structures promoted; (3) the ways in which services are organized, maintained, or encouraged, e.g., informal care arrangements; and (4) the amount of new resources required. In a sense, these represent "alternative futures"; that is, choice among them is determined not only by policy preferences and anticipated outcomes, but by judgments as to the feasibility of each within alternative expectations of future economic and political situations.

The first alternative is to pursue a policy of *improvement of existing long-term-care resources* by making modest changes in current programs. The basic premise of this direction is that, at least in the short term, major structural changes in the financing and delivery of long-term-care services are unlikely to occur, owing to budget constraints and unresolved concerns about the appropriate role of the federal government. There are, however, obvious deficiencies in the major programs now providing long-term-care services (particularly programs supporting home health care and in-home services), which can be remedied through more modest legislative and administrative reforms as well as research and demonstration strategies.

The second alternative follows an opposite premise and asserts that *long-term care requires a separate federal long-term-care benefit program to be coordinated with, but separate from, existing programs.* This line of reasoning assumes that the quality of coordination necessary to make existing resources responsive to long-term-care needs is unlikely to occur in the context of incremental reforms. Long-term care will not acquire the necessary priority, or the necessary political clout in competition for resources, unless there is a clearly identified federal long-term-care initiative. This initiative would be created by federal legislation, and mandated nationwide or made optional with strong financial incentives for state and local participation.

The third alternative requires still another change in orientation. It can be described as an *income strategy for the development of adequate long-term-care resources.* This direction would entail the provision of additional income, or supplemental "buying powers," to individuals who are determined by some criterion to need long-term-care services. Like the second alternative, this requires a major new federal effort, but this direction explicitly attempts to locate as many as possible of the decisions about the nature, quantity, and mix of resources for long-term care with the consumer. It should be noted that this option would most probably have to be combined with other federal efforts to promote and regulate the availability and quality of services, but this option is discussed primarily for its emphasis on the role of the individual in choosing his or her own methods and providers of care.

The fourth major direction is defined broadly as *private-sector-based long-term-care initiatives*. Instead of assuming that the public sector (federal, state, or local) should take the dominant role in creating long-term-care supports and systems of care, this alternative is based on the premise that this responsibility is more appropriately, or more feasibly, located in the private sector. Private sector here is used broadly to include voluntary nonprofit, profit-making, and individual efforts that are not under the auspices of government. In one sense, this direction and the initiatives which logically flow from it represent the most significant departure from current policy trends. This alternative would require a reversal of our increasingly typical assumption that government should bear the responsibility for new social welfare programs.

Most of the specific program suggestions that have emerged from interest groups, Congress, state legislatures, and community agencies can be categorized within one of these four alternatives, but it is important first to debate the broad directions, rather than the specific programmatic manifestations of these directions. Only in this way can the questions of public role and responsibility as well as the inherent value choices be made explicit. Having made decisions on those issues, we can then determine the more concrete and strategic directions required for implementation of these directions.

It is important to recognize that elements of each of these alternatives are compatible with elements of other alternatives. For example, the need for more private-sector involvement in long-term-care strategies is a principle that should help to guide long-term-care development. It is possible to have an increased private-sector role in long-term-care policy, without giving it the central role it holds in the fourth alternative. At this point, we turn to a more extended analysis of each of the four alternatives.

A. Improvement in Existing
Long-Term-Care Programs

The rationale for improving existing programs is that current knowledge in the field, combined with likely budgetary constraints, provides an insufficient basis for proposing options for major structural changes in long-term-care financing, organization, and delivery. Instead, improvements can be made in current programs which will begin to address some of the problems of restricted access, inadequate resources for in-home and community services, and lack of sufficient quality controls. From the standpoint of strategy, this direction explicitly calls for incremental changes and redeployment of existing funding sources. The purpose of these changes is to boost the capacity for each funding source to respond more equitably to long-term-care needs, or to increase the access of individuals to existing long-term-care services. Many such changes have been advanced in the past three years, usually as alterations to Medicaid and Medicare and Title XX. The most complete compendium of such changes was the home health report submitted to the Congress by HHS in October 1979,[36] which proposes legislative and administrative changes in three areas: (1) to increase access to services and provide them in the least restrictive environment; (2) to enhance the quality of existing services; and (3) to improve the efficiency of the existing delivery system. For example, specific legislative and administrative recommendations include:

1. Removing the three-day prior institutionalization requirements for eligibility for home health care benefits under Part A of Medicare.
2. Allowing those states without medically needy programs to provide Medicaid coverage for certain low-income aged, blind, and disabled individuals who need in-home services but are not categorically eligible.
3. Permitting reimbursement for physician assistants and nurse practitioners for review of home health care patient plans under Medicaid or Medicare in rural, medically underserved or health manpower shortage areas.
4. Authorizing the secretary of HHS to establish minimum reimbursement levels for home health benefits under Medicaid.
5. Promoting the development of quality assurance mechanisms for Title XX in-home services.
6. Upgrading the skill requirements for all homemaker/home health aides as a condition of participation in Titles XVIII and XIX.

A focus of incremental change strategies is the past and current long-term-care research and demonstration efforts which emphasize improved coordination and utilization of existing resources with limited "gap-filling" generation of new resources. The principle of better coordination has been the premise of long-term-care demonstration projects over the past ten years, and has become one of the guiding principles of the channeling demonstrations to be financed by HHS over the next several years.[37] Arguments have been made that this approach is the most efficient, making maximum use of existing resources, redeploying them as necessary, or assigning new priorities in the allocation of funds. It is also argued that this is sound policy because it avoids the trap of duplicating support systems that are already in place. Perhaps most importantly in times of fiscal constraint, this direction can be said to be a low-cost option. Rather than create a new long-term-care program, it only marshalls existing long-term-care resources more effectively. Rather than launching major new expenditure programs for long-term care, it puts into place a coordinating or channeling mechanism of some kind. (We should note, however, that cost estimates of this approach vary widely, and there are few data to substantiate any cost estimates to date.)

Questions remain about the wisdom of this course of action. Although in some senses it is a "least change" alternative and perhaps more easily accomplished in the short run, past efforts to coordinate major social systems have not been markedly successful. Even on a limited demonstration basis, attempts to integrate services, or obtain long-lasting coordination of categorical programs, have proven difficult. Callahan makes this point in this paper, as he reviews the track record of demonstration efforts in a variety of fields:

> Success in creating permanent structures and processes of coordination and integration appears to be nonexistent except for some specialized programs in rural areas operated by state government. Given that rural areas frequently lack services, success of these projects may reflect the impact of new resources rather than the coordination and integration of existing providers.[38]

This disillusioning record at the local level has a parallel at the federal level. For example, the Joint Funding Simplification Act has been in existence since 1974, with the express purpose of providing a mechanism for meshing federal programs in order to make these programs more efficient for state and local governments. There were inadequacies in the Joint Funding Simplification Act enabling legislation, but it remains true that few attempts have been made to use this vehicle. At the time of reenactment no pressure was mounted to make it a more effective method of integrating federal programs, even on a demonstration basis. It is difficult to review the history of coordination efforts—on the local, state, and federal levels—without being skeptical of a primarily coordinative strategy for long-term care.

The second issue with regard to coordination concerns the degree of control over existing resources. If the conclusion is that a mandate to "coordinate" is by itself insufficient, what clout should this coordinating agent have in order to shape the expenditure and allocation of resources? The literature suggests several answers to this, ranging from a pool of funding sources to delegated decision-making authority residing under the central direction of the coordinating agency. It seems sufficient to assert that without some form of direct financial control, coordination attempts can hope to have little effect on the current operations of the major systems of income maintenance, social services, health care, housing, rehabilitation, and mental health. Each of these current systems operates under its own bureaucratic structure with different federal-state-local intergovernmental relationships, rules, and regulations. The bureaucratic difficulties are complicated by arbitrary professional distinctions which all work together to make the task of coordination extremely difficult.

It is also generally agreed that coordination should not stand on its own and must be accompanied by alteration and expansion of the social support system. Again, the issue here is one of financing. Most the recent recommendations for coordinating strategies attempt to create new financing for social supports. This involves either an increase in public funding for these services, usually routed through the coordinating agency, or a redeployment of existing resources (more difficult, but not impossible, as can be seen in the gradual shift in priorities of OAA funds over the past five years).

A further issue with regard to coordination efforts is one of cost. Because of the limited data generated from past demonstrations, there is little reliable information on the likely cost of launching coordinating mechanisms for long-term care as part of a national strategy. The Federal Council on Aging, in its 1978 report on the frail elderly, made an attempt to estimate this cost, assuming a series of coordinating agencies staffed by case managers and performing the functions of diagnosis, assessment, coordination of services, and monitoring of client progress. Their estimate was in the range of $0.7 to $1.7 billion for the frail elderly only. These estimates are based on average cost per client, per year of $1,000 for case management services.[39] These costs are estimates solely of the coordination function, not of the expansion of social supports which are believed to be a necessary accompaniment. If these estimates have any validity, even as rough guides to true cost, it is clear that the low-cost nature of this alternative must be seriously questioned. Under the guise of coordination, we may be contemplating a major new direct service which, by all accounts, is highly professionalized, specialized, and likely to be costly. There is a certain irony that this highly professionalized mode of service is the solution to a problem which arises from the need by many for assistance with the mundane tasks of daily living.

The program initiatives which have been suggested to improve coordination are several. Most prominent now is HHS's channeling demonstration program. Further, the Older Americans Act and its new regulations move toward the concept of a coordinating agency. This concept was always inherent in the "area agency" design, but has proven difficult to implement in many, if not most, local areas. It is only since 1973 that the federal government has been urging the Area Agencies on Aging (AAAs) to take on more direct and specific coordinating functions over service delivery (as opposed to direct service provision, planning, and fund allocation). This can be seen in the new regulations. Even so, the use of AAAs as coordinating agencies in long-term care remains, from the standpoint of federal policy, more a theory than widespread practice.

However, several states on their own have taken steps to make AAAs a type of coordinating agency. Pennsylvania and Massachusetts have perhaps the longest-standing programs in which local area agencies act as planners and brokers for the service plans of individuals, using available service entitlements and supplementing these benefit programs with Older Americans Act funds as necessary. In Philadelphia, for example, the AAA acts as a case manager and controls Title XX resources in addition to OAA funds. Illinois has moved in this direction as well, having appropriated over $9 million per year specifically for community-based social support services to be dispensed by AAAs as part of a statewide program of community-based long-term care.

Other proposals which fall within this incremental alternative include suggestions for increasing Title III Social Services funding under the Older Americans Act in order to provide greater local resources for in-home and community supports and recommendations for administrative action on developing common service definitions and standards for in-home care now provided under Titles XVIII, XIX, XX, and the OAA.

In general, all of the incremental changes included in this first policy direction can be viewed as first steps in a phased process of change. Unfortunately, such changes are often proposed independently of overall systems change and with no view toward further reforms. While minor program improvements may reduce some of the current disincentives for providing in-home services, the basic financing for long-term-care service would remain unchanged and would continue to flow primarily through the medical care system.

On the other hand, the advantage of this approach is that change can be accomplished gradually and at low cost. As the least-change option, it may be the most politically feasible at the moment.

B. A New Federal Benefit Program for Long-Term Care

The second approach to federal long-term-care policy is to create a new benefit program that would consolidate existing financial support for long-term care and expand federal responsibility for noninstitutional long-term care. The rationale for this approach is that existing federal

methods for financing long-term care—normally, Medicare and Medicaid—were not designed to provide coverage for noninstitutional care.
Thus, the medical and institutional biases of these funding sources are
likely to remain, despite small changes made in their benefit structure.
Therefore, major new legislation is required if long-term-care financing is
to be successfully redirected.

This approach is not new. Several attempts have been made or are
under way to develop federal long-term-care legislation. In the following
analysis these past efforts are used as examples to illustrate some of the
policy issues posed by this approach.

The first purpose of all proposed new federal long-term-care programs
has been expansion of federal responsibility and financing for noninstitutional long-term-care services. For example, the Medicare Long Term
Care Act of 1979 (H.R. 58, often referred to as the Conable Bill), authorized federal funding for many community-based services, as well as
community long-term-care centers which would function as coordinating
agencies. The bill was unusual in that it provided financing for institutional care as well, without revoking any existing federal authorities
for such care. This federal authority was proposed as a new Part D of
Medicare.

Most other proposed legislation has focused exclusively on noninstitutional care. An example was the recently debated Title XXI of the Social
Security Act, which had as its purpose the creation of one comprehensive
title within the act that could centralize the authorizations for noninstitutional long-term-care services now included under Titles XVIII, XIX, and
XX. Authorized services included in-home nursing care, physical,
speech, and occupational therapy, home health aide services, adult day
care services, respite care services, and assessment and screening.

The methods proposed for financing services under a new federal program have varied. For example, the Conable Bill proposed grants to
states. Money was designated for the purposes of community-based care,
but decisions on the expenditure of funds were delegated to state or local
government. This approach falls midway between "block grant" financing and a more specific categorical long-term-care program. The proposed
Title XXI had more complex financing, using the Medicare model of
third-party reimbursement. Clients were required first to exhaust a prescribed amount of services for which a copayment mechanism is trig-
gred, until a ceiling amount per individual is reached; one hundred
percent federal financing is then resumed for costs above that ceiling. A
third approach was taken by the Medicaid Community Care Act of 1980,
H.R. 6194 (the Pepper-Waxman Bill), which raised the federal financial
participation under Medicaid by 25 percentage points up to a maximum of
90 percent federal financial participation (FFP) for states expanding the

availability of community care according to the provisions of the legislation.

Financing of long-term care is usually not the only purpose of these new federal programs. Most examples of this approach attempt to change the long-term-care delivery system as well. Typically, a coordinating agency is suggested, in order to ensure that services are more responsive to individual need. Plans for this coordinating agency take different forms. Title XXI required that governors designate a lead state agency (health, or welfare, or aging agency) to work with other state agencies in establishing local Preadmission Screening Assessment Teams (PATs). These teams were to have case management responsibilities, including evaluation of the functional capabilities of each individual; development of a plan of care; assistance in obtaining needed services; and so forth. The Conable Bill envisioned that similar functions would be performed by the community long-term-care centers to be established under the bill. These centers were to be given payment authority, as well as responsibility for service provision and service coordination, and thus represented a potent new agent in the long-term-care delivery system. The Pepper-Waxman Bill similarly called for an assessment and coordinating function, in this case to be carried out under the authority of the state Medicaid agency. In effect, most bills which pursue the approach of establishing a new federal benefit program also establish a new delivery system at the state and local levels, superimposing this on the existing delivery system.

New federal benefit programs for long-term care could be designed to include more than the range of community-based health and social services which are authorized by the legislation cited above. Greater reliance could be placed on creative housing and supportive living arrangements as the hub around which long-term-care services could be focused. HUD has been only minimally involved to date in the long-term-care policy process, but is beginning to consider more seriously congregate living arrangements and renovation of existing housing to meet the needs of the functionally impaired. An example of HUD's growing involvement is a national program using special Section 8 set-asides which would require private developers to work with state and local health, welfare, social service, and aging agencies to integrate social supports with housing construction. This represents an explicit attempt to target new federal benefits to meet long-term-care housing needs, an area that has been so often ignored.

The choice of a new benefit program as the preferred federal long-term care strategy raises several issues. The first, and perhaps most basic, is whether a new categorical program will further fragment the provision of long-term care, or whether it provides the much-needed federal authority for financing noninstitutional care. To understand this issue, it is necessary to recall that most proposals for new benefit programs include weak provisions for integrating the new system with existing programs. The lack of integration is threefold: (1) the financing of community-based care is often not well related to institutional and noninstitutional care; (2) the methods for delivering institutional and noninstitutional care are often uncoordinated; and (3) there are limited provisions for common eligibility definitions across programs.

With regard to financing, for example, there is no incentive in the new program proposals for a trade-off or substitution of noninstitutional for institutional costs. With regard to the delivery system, some of the new programs provide for coordinating agencies, but these organizations can exist with little relationship to organizations already mandated to perform some of the same coordination functions (for example, PSROs, AAAs, and health services agencies or HSA). In fairness, some of the new programs include language encouraging coordination among all these actors, but none is persuasive that the new system for providing community-based long-term care is not duplicative of existing organizational structures.

These problems are inherent in a new benefit program. In any such approach which provides a major new federal benefit the trade-off is the increased visibility and authority provided to the defined program, versus the acknowledged risk of creating yet another program which may become difficult to control, and which does not replace but merely adds to existing programmatic authorities.

Thus, a strategic decision is necessary in reviewing this policy direction. The degree to which one advocates a new benefit program is likely to depend on one's sense of the likelihood, under existing financial and program structures, of overcoming the present medical and institutional bias. The changes proposed in Medicaid and Medicare to improve access to noninstitutional services can be viewed as small-scale program revisions with little chance of reversing current patterns of care. Although such changes may increase overall access to community-based care, they inherently continue service financing in a medical context, consistent with the medical model of their legislative bases. A new approach, although categorical, can set new priorities and has some hope of overcoming the predominance of medical and institutional care. It is important to note, however, that several of the proposed new benefit programs are built on the Medicare model and incorporate fee-for-service reimbursements which may prove as cost inflationary as existing health care programs.

With respect to intergovernmental relations, a new federal benefit program obviously assumes a greater role in the financing and direction of long-term care services. Any of these proposals will directly alter the balance of federal-state-local relationships. A presumed goal of this approach is greater uniformity across states and a more visible federal presence in priority and standard setting. Proposals like the Conable Bill also delineate greater responsibilities at the state and local levels for coordination and service delivery.

The relationship of a new federal benefit program to existing informal supports is unclear. All of the programs advanced to date seem to encourage the increasing professionalization of community-based long-term care. The Conable Bill and the proposed Title XXI continue funding primarily to provider agencies, with little explicit encouragement of informal/familial modes of care. This affects the cost of services as well as the quality and nature of service. Overprofessionalization is a real risk in the expansion of community-based care. The new benefit program approach does nothing to reduce this risk, and, in fact, seems to promote it. Dollars ultimately end up in the hands of providers. Further, none of the proposals speaks directly about ways of supporting families and informal networks. Several include respite care as a new benefit, a service which is often regarded as a necessary complement to a family's willingness and ability to provide long-term care to a chronically impaired person. The concern still exists, however, that an expanded federal program of long-term benefits will erode rather than support existing informal care. Without provisions to ensure that family care systems are supported, it can be argued that they may in fact be reduced.

Strategically, precedent indicates that a new categorical definition of noninstitutional care is more likely to attract the legislative attention and budgetary appropriations necessary to expand care resources. The pattern of development of domestic social welfare programs shows that categorical definition and separation of programs yield accelerated interest group support, professional advocacy, and financing.

The failure to enact any of the legislation described above, or similar legislation, stems from three causes: no definitive knowledge of what expanded community-based long-term care is likely to cost;[40] little Congressional confidence in the ability of community-based delivery systems to ration or monitor effectively the utilization (and thus cost) of expanded long-term care; and no constituency yet organized to support such legislation.

Suspicion of the potential high cost of community-based long-term care is likely to continue. As Pollak and Greenberg state in chapter 7, below, research on long-term-care costs is characterized more by good intentions than by significant results. There are few data on either the average cost of community-based long-term care or expected utilization. It is hoped that HHS's proposed channeling demonstration will emphasize the need for better cost data. However, the difficulties in obtaining necessary data are well recognized, and it seems unlikely that data to answer the policy question will be available for at least three to five years. In fact, Pollak and Greenberg suggest that it will more likely take ten years and a considerable amount of money to obtain good cost data from demonstration experiments.[41]

Given this uncertainty about cost, it is understandable that the financing methods proposed for most new federal benefit programs are grant-in-aid approaches. Grants-in-aid provide the federal government with greater control over total expenditures than would, for example, an entitlement approach. Even so, the fear remains that any new program for community-based long-term care will soon create demand for much more extensive financing of this care. In the present Congressional mood of fiscal restraint, this could be an insurmountable strategic barrier to this approach.

Congressional concern about the capacity of existing service delivery systems to provide long-term care effectively is reflected in the presence of new delivery mechanisms in each bill discussed in this paper. The intent is to create a new control point on long-term-care expenditures in order to avoid the rapidly escalating costs that occurred under Medicaid. Knowledge about coordinating agencies is almost as scarce as cost data. Although the value of "channeling" and case management agencies is now often assumed, it can be argued that these agencies result in merely another level of organizational ineptitude and consequent cost. We do not debate the issue here. Callahan states the arguments for and against such agencies in chapter 5. It seems sufficient to note that, as of now, there is no evidence that such agencies, launched nationwide, would contribute benefits that would offset their cost.

C. An Income Strategy to Ensure Provision of Long-Term Care

The distinguishing characteristic of an income strategy for securing adequate long-term care for those in need is the control it gives over financial resources to consumers of care. In this sense, the approaches discussed so far are service strategies; that is, they expand the availability, or reorient the balance, of long-term-care services. The purposes of those approaches are to ensure adequate services and guarantee that the services are appropriately matched with individuals in need.

By contrast, the income strategy seeks to give people the resources to obtain care for themselves. From a federal perspective, this strategy changes the flow of benefits. The typical dollar flow—from government to provider to person in need—changes to: government to person in need to provider. This change affects policy and programs, and we believe it reflects profound differences of values concerning the nature of government responsibility and on individual autonomy.

Income strategies for long-term care take two forms. The first and most obvious is the direct, cash supplementation of income for a functionally impaired person, in an amount necessary to pay for costs of care required by reason of impairment. This income is provided over and above basic living costs, which are met (in theory, at least) by Social Security, SSI, and other income assistance.

A second type of income strategy is the use of vouchers to pay for long-term care. In this option, the benefit is provided not in the form of cash, but in an alternative "currency" that can be used only for long-term care. The voucher mechanism is a more restricted benefit. Whereas cash can be used to obtain goods and services other than long-term care if the beneficiary so chooses, the voucher limits buying power to long-term care. Although the differences between cash and vouchers are significant, we first discuss the policy choices and assumptions which underlie both mechanisms.

A basic assumption of both cash and voucher strategies is that government can somehow define—and *should* define—an entitlement to long-term care. Entitlement denotes a benefit that must be given to every person meeting predefined eligibility criteria. Precedents here are the income support programs: Social Security, Aid for Dependent Children (AFDC), SSI, and disability insurance. Entitlements to care, particularly medical care, also exist; Medicaid and Medicare are closely related examples.

Establishing a long-term-care entitlement would represent a major assumption of federal responsibility for long-term care. Even if the entitlement were narrowly defined—for example, by adding a small increment to SSI benefits for individuals over age 75, as suggested in the staff report to the Federal Council on Aging Task Force on the Frail Elderly—the precedent thereby established could be far-reaching. Limited benefits under an entitlement program would establish a precedent of federal government legal and fiscal responsibility for the functionally impaired. The degree of this responsibility could be debated, but the point we highlight here is the new federal responsibility entailed in the extension of such an entitlement.

The most probable way to extend a cash benefit would be supplementation of an existing income support system. These systems already have judicial interpretation on the nature of the entitlement which they confer. Extension of these programs to include a long-term-care cash supplement would carry with it the weight of these precedents. A voucher could be implemented through a new system—even, perhaps, a service-oriented system. For example, long-term-care vouchers could be issued by AAAs to all individuals meeting a standardized test of disability. If this mechanism were used, the entitlement to care would be less clear, because of the discretion likely in awarding voucher amounts and the probable lack of uniformity in the program administration.

A second major principle underlying the income approach is the value given to individual autonomy in the choice of services. In general, the income strategies seek to maximize client choice and control over service benefits. There are two main reasons for providing benefits in cash rather than in the form of services. The first, and we believe the major, reason is to give people capacity to make their own decisions on utilization of resources. The second reason, we believe, has to do with economic efficiencies; but this is discussed at a later point. The implicit assumption is that individuals in need should whenever possible choose who provides assistance and the scope and nature of the assistance.

The impairment of many consumers will require that functionally impaired persons have recourse to assistance in obtaining help in the choice of long-term care services. For example, most voucher strategies incorporate a case management structure that is available to a recipient at his/her discretion. Yet, the primary goal is to have decisions made more fully by individuals and families, with government limitation of choice only as necessary to prevent exploitation, fraud, and abuse.

Income strategies affect provision of services. These strategies carry with them an implicit "market model" of services. Resources to purchase services are made available; the client then chooses, on the market, the services or benefits he/she wishes to purchase. When cash is provided, a pure market approach is present. When a voucher plan is used, a modified market principle is in operation. For example, in the Illinois long-term-care voucher experiment, voucher use is limited to a defined set of services, but the choice of providers of services is not circumscribed. Purchase from informal and family providers of care is allowable. In the voucher models described by Pollak, vouchers are also limited to long-term-care services. However, Pollak adds an interesting variation, proposing that the case management agency which could assist the client be viewed as a service resource like any other. That is, the client should have choice among alternative case management agencies. This recognizes an important point in the use of a voucher system; any mechanism established to advise or "help" a client is likely to introduce procedures that reduce the client's free choice. Pollak's idea of competitive case management systems is a useful offset to this tendency.

The market principle in service delivery also has implications for the use of family supports. The income strategies under discussion here can lead naturally to subsidizing family and informal care. Given free rein in the use of funds for long-term care, people would likely choose to finance care through relatives, friends, and other informal providers. This is presumably of benefit to the client, in that it encourages care from people who know the client and have an emotional attachment to him. It has the further benefit of providing income to those who perform the care. (This point should not be overstated. There is little evidence regarding choices that people would make in spending money for long-term care. Many might prefer the more business-like arrangements of agency-based care, preferring to avoid issues of dependency that may arise from care solely by relatives or friends.) In any case, the policy goal of supporting informal care providers is more directly accomplished through an income strategy than through any other approach.

An income strategy by itself involves the federal government more heavily in the direct financing of long-term care and further removes it from questions of resource creation and service delivery. Issues of developing service delivery systems and coordinating mechanisms are left to either free enterprise or state and local government. In fact, one could question whether a pure income strategy obviates the need for any federal role in service delivery. It is equally likely that an income strategy would not be feasible without more explicit public responsibility for standard setting in order to protect the consumer against fraud, abuse, and low-quality services.

The experience with income strategies for long-term care is limited. The Veterans Administration operates a small aid and attendant program which provides cash benefits to eligible veterans to purchase their own care. Since 1958, California has supplemented incomes of impaired individuals to allow them to purchase attendant care ($400 per month for the moderately impaired; $600 per month for the severely disabled). Approximately 60 to 70 percent of recipients purchase their care from family members. California's experience indicates some difficulties in such a system; there have been recurrent complaints of misuses of funds, overpayment and overcharging, and inadequate quality of care. As a result, legislation is pending to convert this system to one with more provider agency control. On the other hand, the advantages are also clear. Individuals do choose their own providers; the system is implemented with little administrative overhead; and family support seems to have been retained.

In sum, income strategies for long-term care represent a policy direction which follows naturally upon the precedent of income assistance for the aged and disabled, but which differs sharply from current trends toward expanded service strategies. Adopting such a strategy requires a substantial federal commitment of finances, as well as a clearer definition of federal responsibility than is required by any other approach to expansion of long-term care.

D. Encouragement of Private-Sector Responses to Long-Term Needs

The fourth direction for a future policy requires some prefacing comments. Encouraging private-sector initiatives in long-term care does not exclude the three approaches already discussed. Private-sector initiatives are compatible with those approaches. In fact, as we stated earlier, all approaches should seek to promote private-sector involvement. (We use private sector here to denote efforts of families and private individuals, as well as private voluntary agency and corporate sectors.) As an example, we have pointed out the implications of an income strategy for securing the involvement of families and other private, informal providers of care.

However, it is possible to conceive of policy directions for long-term care in which the federal government plays a supporting or enabling role, but in which major responsibility for financing and service provision is shared with the private sector. In general, these approaches to long-term care have been less well conceived and less carefully defined. The preponderance of literature on future directions is devoted to government-based approaches, consistent with the growing pressures and emerging demand that long-term care should be a public responsibility. However, the chapters below, particularly chapter 5 by Callahan and chapter 6 by Fullerton, suggest ideas for private-sector action which we believe are sufficiently intriguing and thought provoking to warrant further study. We first review the models suggested by Fullerton and Callahan, and then discuss implications of these models for federal policy.

Fullerton suggests a financing option for long term care with the following elements:

1. Voluntary establishment of individual long-term-care accounts. Payments of two percent of taxable income up to a maximum of $1,000 per year could be made into a private account by anyone aged 40 or older. The first $250 of this account would count as a tax credit; the remainder could be used as a tax deduction.

2. Expenditures could be made from the account only after reaching age 65, and only to purchase a defined set of long-term-care services or for private insurance policies covering nursing home services. Nursing home insurance would be regulated by an effective system (backed up by fiscal incentives, if possible) for determining need for care, and by government involvement in setting nursing home rates.

3. Medicaid would be amended to mandate the same federally defined set of long-term-care services to all Medicaid eligibles over 75, and all SSI recipients eligible on the basis of disability.

4. A national lottery would be established to raise $20 billion in the first year of operation, of which one-half would be used to finance program benefits.

5. The remaining half of lottery revenues would go to states to develop long-term-care resources.

6. Social Security benefits for those aged 75 and older would be increased five percent.[42]

Fullerton's option is a financing method which encourages and relies on private investment, avoiding new taxes for purposes of long-term care (except as Medicaid and Social Security benefits would expand).

Callahan proposes a service delivery option which encourages private-sector involvement, particularly consumer involvement.[43] He terms this the "association of users" model. It would create a nonprofit organization of users (children and their parents, elderly, handicapped) which would recruit members of the population group at risk, and receive federal recognition as a service entity. These groups would negotiate packages of service with local providers, provide case management services for members unable to do so on their own, and work with federal and state governments to eliminate red tape and eligibility barriers. The organization of users would not control payment for service, but could control the flow of patients who are members.

The direction suggested by these approaches is one in which government responsibility is reduced, although certainly not eliminated. In the Callahan option, for example, a primary government role is still assumed in the financing and allocation of long-term-care dollars, but consumers have a more direct voice and active role with regard to provider agencies. In the Fullerton model, a major part of the federal responsibility for long-term care shifts to individuals and families although the federal government remains responsible for financing care for the poor.

Ultimately, these and similar options differ from the other approaches in their view of the appropriate role of the federal, state, and local governments in long-term care. These options assume that government should first be supportive of private and individual initiatives. The implication is that only when these break down should full government control be the preferred option.

Advocacy of these options can grow from several rationales. Private-sector initiatives can be supported because of a belief that individuals and families should retain responsibility and control over their own care; because of a political ideology that prefers private-sector rather than public-sector initiatives; or merely because of strategic considerations —i.e., an assumption that public responsibility is unlikely to be extended to long-term care in the near future.

The advantages of these options are clear, and are discussed by Fullerton and Callahan in their respective papers. Most of the advantages derive from the increased responsibility given to individuals and families. Some disadvantages can also be identified.

The main argument against reliance on a private-sector-based strategy is that there is little likelihood that private initiatives would result in the development of financing arrangements or services adequate to meet the needs of low-income individuals. The historical failure of the private sector to provide adequate insurance to fill gaps in Medicare coverage, or the documented abuses of privately owned long-term-care institutions, are reasons that some analysts remain wary of private-sector efforts not monitored by the public sector.

The intent here, and the intent of the two authors cited above, is not to advance specific proposals, but to stimulate more consideration of options involving the private sector. At a minimum, the policy decisions likely to be made in setting up public-sector options should be reviewed against criteria that examine the possibility of greater private-sector initiative.

V. Recommendations for Change

The long-term-care policy debate has too often faltered at the juncture of moving from analysis to recommendations. The problems are so varied, our knowledge of impacts so limited, the costs of any proposed changes so high that it is easy to understand why analysts have difficulty in agreeing on recommendations for change. Despite these uncertainties, we believe that there is a clear need to alter the basic structures which govern the provision of long-term-care services and that specific proposals must be put forward and debated. This paper therefore concludes with a series of recommendations on basic parameters of a long-term-care system, followed by a preferred strategy for change.

The first three recommendations address need and eligibility for long-term care. First, the target population for long-term-care services should be linked to a demonstrated need for care based on the presence of functional limitation. Functional limitation—that is, the inability to perform activities of daily living necessary for self-care and self-support—is the most basic and generic indicator for need for the population at risk. Use of this criterion of need represents a movement away from medical diagnosis as the primary determinant of eligibility for long-term-care services, and thus is a step toward the demedicalization of the long-term-care system.

A second recommendation is that there be no arbitrary age cutoff for eligibility for publicly supported long-term care. This is based on the demographic analysis of need, which indicates equal numbers of impaired persons above and below the arbitrary eligibility point of age 65. It is also based on a recognition that age has not proven to be an accurate predictor of need in many respects. Further, we believe it would be shortsighted to develop a system of care of impaired elderly persons which could not be easily adapted to meet the needs of younger impaired persons. With regard to this issue, a distinction between an ideal long-term-care system and the interim stages necessary to achieve that system is useful. In developing financial and service resources for long-term care, it may be necessary to begin with adults over age 65 in order to build on the structure and political popularity of current benefit programs. However, the longer-range goal of a service system responsive to all impaired adults should be explicit.

The third recommendation is that access to care should be equitably distributed to persons of all income levels. Again, the distinction between an ideal system and stages necessary to achieve this complete system is useful. The preference is to make services available to persons at all income levels, but it is clear that resource levels now and in the foreseeable future will require targeting of public funds to pay for needed care. Thus, for the immediate future, public policy should continue to direct subsidies of long-term care first to low-income individuals. As a matter of strategy, it is probably more feasible to expand benefits for this most needy population, and then work toward coverage for higher income levels at a later period.

Our fourth recommendation calls for expanded availability of social and other supports to provide a more appropriate and cost-effective balance to existing medical care services and providers. The long-term-care service system should give a more prominent role to social supports within a system that includes the following major types of assistance:

1. Adequate income, sufficient to meet basic needs.
2. Social supports, including activities that substitute for or replace lost abilities to perform day-to-day tasks necessary for independent living.
3. Health care, including primary care, acute care, and continuing care for chronic conditions, in either an institutional or a noninstitutional setting.
4. Adequate housing, including housing arrangements which in themselves minimize or facilitate the replacement of lost capacities.

Social supports should explicitly include familial and other informal supports. If personal care services related to long-term care become the exclusive province of professionally administered, formal agencies, care could become more expensive than it need be, and also less closely related to the preferences of impaired people.

With regard to the organizaton and delivery of long-term-care services, it is clear that no one model for service delivery is sufficiently well documented to warrant a uniform federal prescription of service arrangements. Decisions on service delivery systems should remain the responsibility of state and local governments and private agencies. Federal policy should seek only to ensure that the basic elements of long-term-care service provision—income supports, social supports, health care, and housing arrangements—are made available in ways that allow for response to diverse individual needs and conditions. It is hoped that the recently funded federally sponsored "channeling" demonstrations will provide new knowledge about the costs and effectiveness of several models of service delivery. However, the findings of these projects should be considered in conjunction with the outcomes of other "natural" experiments now under way in states and localities before final choices are made among delivery systems. A central agency to plan, arrange, coordinate, and monitor long-term-care services may have to be made available for many people, but other individuals and families may not need the intervention of another professional to perform these functions. We need expanded knowledge of alternative methods for service delivery before federal policy should promote one rather than another.

In the context of the recommendations discussed above, we turn now to our preferred direction for change, which is based primarily on a broadened federal income strategy supported by expanded service and resource development. Income support must underlie any long-term-care service program, and the primary federal responsibility can best be met through the provision of additional income or buying power which will enable individuals and their families to purchase needed long-term-care services. This strategy seeks to maximize individual autonomy, and it reduces government responsibility for decisions on the specific types of care an individual needs and receives.

Our notion of an income strategy does not rest on any single new federal income entitlement, but rather, on a modification of income support systems currently in place. Already SSI and Social Security affect more persons in need of long-term care than any other federal programs. We would modify these two programs and then turn to tax credits and private pensions for further assistance.

With respect to SSI, optional provisions governing the use of supplementary payments for the purchase of domiciliary care and other supported housing could be expanded. This would use the purchasing power of income supplements to create a demand for alternative living arrangements. Current provisions for financing domiciliary care would need to be modified with the possible addition of provisions for quality control and standard setting as part of the SSI payment system.

A second change which could be pursued through the SSI system is a supplemental payment, based on disability, for attendant care. In most states where this is now done, as in California, the supplemental payment is financed by state Title XX funds, not SSI funds. However, a supplement for severe disability could be made a federal SSI provision with full federal financing, or a required state matching payment could be set at a rate more favorable to the state than the costs of institutional care.

Another component of an income strategy could be to make provision in the Social Security benefit structure for an additional payment for persons over age 75 or 80. The incidence of disability among this age group is sufficiently high to warrant additional funds to pay for needed aids for daily living. For many people, these funds would enable them to continue to live in their communities in an independent or supportive housing arrangement.

Another component of an income strategy would be tax credits to families who care for persons with functional impairments. The purpose is to eliminate current financial disincentives for providing such care, which can be most easily accomplished through the tax system. Use of tax credits allows relief to middle class families who bear a heavy burden of care, but often receive no assistance from public programs.

A final component of the income strategy is expanded use of private pensions. Additional incentives for pension creation could be developed along the lines suggested by Fullerton in chapter 6, below, or through other provisions. There is a growing interest on the part of private insurance companies in this type of solution.

The advantages of an income strategy are several: (1) it preserves individual autonomy and control over long-term-care decisions; (2) it can be accomplished through modification of existing systems, and so its implementation problems are less severe than if it had required an entirely new categorical federal budget or uniform service delivery system; (3) it provides strong incentives for the preservation and use of informal supports; and (4) it relies heavily on the private sector and provides financial incentives for private-sector initiatives in long-term care, thus stimulating improvements in long-term-care service supply.

In proposing an income strategy as the primary direct federal responsibility, we are no less aware of the need for expanded service development and resource creation. Providing impaired individuals with the funds to purchase care is effective only if services are available to be bought. However, the development of services and service delivery systems should not be the centerpiece of federal long-term-care policy. Instead, the federal role in service provision should concentrate on (1) testing the utility of different types of services, and (2) promoting resource development and creation in areas where services are scarce. This is particularly important in many rural areas of the nation. If federal activity is focused on research, demonstration, and resource development activities, the federal role with regard to services is complementary with and supportive of the income strategy.

A third aspect of the recommended strategy concerns housing. Housing is perhaps the most ignored aspect of long-term-care policy development despite the critical importance of expanding the availability of supportive and other housing alternatives. In addition to encouraging congregate care through SSI, the preferred federal role here is again developmental. Experimentation with different kinds of housing alternatives is best accomplished by federal developmental assistance and provision of incentives to the private sector to promote expanded service-linked housing arrangements.

Finally, although we have not specifically addressed it, our strategy implies a continued public role in standard setting. Regulatory policy may need some review and streamlining, but the recommendation of an income strategy with a supportive service component does not imply a significantly diminished governmental responsibility for quality assurance.

VI. Conclusion

As the policy debate moves on, increased attention will be given to the appropriate balance of responsibility among various public agencies, among the different levels of government, and between government and the private sector. In this chapter, we have suggested several different ways in which the federal role could be developed, and have recommended one as preferable within the existing constraints on policy and program development.

The strategy outlined here recommends emphasis at the federal level on the provision of income to enable those in need of long-term care to secure such care. This strategy does not deny the importance of the other basic elements of long-term care. However, it recognizes that the federal role can best be expressed through use of the major income maintenance and tax programs already identified as federal responsibilities and which are efficiently administered at the federal level. We have urged that state and local governments maintain and expand their responsibilities for service delivery. Significant improvements in the coordination and organization of services are possible, and the federal government should continue to test and demonstrate improvements which could then be incorporated in state and local programs. Finally, we have argued that the federal government should provide incentives for local and private-sector initiatives in the critical long-term-care component of housing.

Although we believe that this strategy provides a framework for the development of future policy, it is important to emphasize a more pressing point. Whichever alternative is chosen, improvements in long-term-care policy should begin at once. The nature of the need, both now and in the future, requires short-term as well as longer-term response by the public and private sectors. This sense of urgency should underlie any choices, and must not be lost in the complexity of the policy debate.

Notes

1. See chapter 4, below.

2. Bernice Neugarten, "Policy for the 1980's: Age or Need Entitlement?" *National Journal Issues Book,* Washington, D.C., November, 1979.

3. It should be noted that the definition can appropriately incorporate disabled children who have need for long-term-care services. We exclude them from the purview of this paper because the kinds of family, community, and institutional supports available differ significantly from those normally available to the adult population. We have, therefore, limited our potential population to adults with needs for long-term-care services.

4. See chapter 5, below, p. 152.

5. For a full discussion of poverty among the elderly, see statement of Mollie Orshansky, Office of Research and Statistics, SSA, before the House Committee on Aging, August 9, 1978.

6. "Public Policy and the Frail Elderly," Staff Report to the Federal Council on Aging. HEW, December, 1978.

7. "Some Prospects for the Future Elderly Population," Statistical Reports of Older Americans, AoA HEW, January, 1978, p. 3.

8. A. Z. Nagi, "An Epidemiology of Disability among Adults in the U.S.," *Millbank Memorial Fund Quarterly* 54:439–67 (1976).

9. National Long Term Care Project Final Report, Center for the Study of Welfare Policy, University of Chicago, August 22, 1980, pp. 11–12.

10. "Long Term Care for the Elderly and Disabled," Budget Issue Paper, Congressional Budget Office, February, 1977, p. xix.

11. Ibid., p. xix.

12. "Entering a Nursing Home—Costly Implications for Medicaid and the Elderly," General Accounting Office, November 24, 1979, p. 5.

13. Rules and Regulations, Grants for State and Community Programs on Aging, 45 CFR 1321.43, March 31, 1980.

14. "Home Health and Other In-Home Services: Titles XVIII, XIX, XX of The Social Security Act," Report to the Congress, HEW, October, 1979.

15. HEW Announcement on Channeling Demonstrations, March 21, 1980.

16. For example, see the list of studies cited by James Callahan, chapter 5, below, p. 179, note 2.

17. See chapter 4, below, p. 143.

18. See chapter 3, below, p. 91.

19. See chapter 5, below, pp. 164–66.

20. See chapter 4, below, p. 129.

21. See chapter 2, below, pp. 63–65.

22. See chapter 4, below, p. 130.

23. See also Callahan, Gisle, Diamond, Morris, "Responsibility of Families for their Severely Disabled Elders," *Health Care Financing Review,* Winter, 1980.

24. See chapter 4, below, p. 133.

25. See chapter 2, below, p. 139. See also fig. 1.

26. See chapter 4, below, p. 126.

27. For a discussion of the impact of inflation and fiscal crisis on future health policy, see Phillip R. Lee, M.D., and Carroll L. Estes, "The Federal Government, Health Policy and Health Care of the Disadvantaged," April 15, 1980.

28. See "Perpetuation of the Poverty Cycle for the Aged," by Richard Lehrman, Staff, U.S. House of Representatives, Select Committee on Aging.

29. Lee and Estes, "The Federal Government, Health Policy and Health Care," p. 59.

30. See chapter 2, below, p. 68.

31. See chapter 5, below, pp. 154–56.

32. Ibid., p. 156.

33. Ibid., p. 155.

34. Carroll Estes, "Social Policies for the Aged in the 1980's," January, 1980, p. 5. (To be published in *Generations*.)

35. "Home Health and Other In-Home Services."

36. Ibid.

37. See ASPE Notice of Intent on LTC Channeling Demonstrations.

38. See chapter 5, below, p. 161.

39. "Public Policy and the Frail Elderly."

40. See chapter 7, below. As Pollak and Greenberg there note, past research and demonstration efforts have not adequately addressed the question of potential demand or expected utilization which is essential to any consideration of costs. See their discussion, pp. 221–22.

41. Ibid., p. 223.

42. See chapter 6, below, pp. 202–7.

43. See chapter 5, below, p. 170.

2

Health and Social Factors Relevant to Long-Term-Care Policy

Lewis H. Butler and Paul W. Newacheck

Introduction and Summary

In this chapter we examine the prevalence of chronic illness and disability among the elderly and the social factors associated with such illness and disability. The purpose is to provide a basis for discussion and debate on how health and social factors should affect future long-term-care policy. The analysis is based primarily on previously unpublished data from the Health Interview Survey and the National Nursing Home Survey.[1] The source and limitations of the survey data are discussed in the appendix to this chapter.

As a starting point we assume that persons who are limited in their ability to carry on their major activity, and especially those who are unable to do so, are potentially in need of noninstitutional and institutional long-term-care services. That is, we define them here as the population potentially at risk. Their total number in the over-65 population is about 8.4 million, of which 3.8 million are unable to conduct their major activity.

The analysis is divided into four parts. In the first, we analyze health status of the elderly by age using three different age groups—65 through 74, 75 through 84, and 85 and over. The data reveal that almost all of the decline in health associated with increasing age is accounted for by chronic rather than acute conditions. Chronic conditions cause about 34 percent of the population aged 65 to 74 to be limited in their ability to carry on their major activity, that is, work outside the home or housework. The proportion rises to about 57 percent in the 85-plus population. About half of those limited in their major activity report that they are *unable* to carry on their major activity. As might be expected, they con-

We would like to express our thanks to a number of persons who assisted in the development of this paper. We are particularly grateful to Aileen Harper for her excellent research assistance in the early stages of the paper. We also appreciate useful comments provided by Gail Bronson, William Clark, Sidney Katz, Mary Grace Kovar, Peter May, the Symposium Steering Committee, and our colleagues at the Health Policy Program.

sume a large share of the medical services used by the elderly. Heart disease, arthritis, and chronic rheumatism are the leading causes of their disability, followed by senility, impairments of the lower extremities and hips, and hypertensive disease.

It is apparent from comparing the prevalence of these conditions, and the resulting disability across age groups, that there is no abrupt decline in health status at 65 or any other particular age. The trend is progressive, becoming apparent in middle age and building steadily up through the 85-plus group. These findings are consistent with prior research and are useful largely in emphasizing that, although the incidence of functional disability increases with age, those at risk are not confined to any particular age group. In fact, nearly half of those reporting that they are unable to carry on their major activity are under 65 (NCHS, 1977a). These findings suggest that using such commonly proposed age thresholds as 65 or 75 in determining eligibility for long-term-care programs may result in excluding a substantial proportion of the population potentially in need of long-term-care services.

In the second section we look at which social factors are associated with the population potentially in need of long-term care. The factors examined are sex, income, race, region of the country, and residence (rural or urban). Since marital status and living arrangements have special significance, those factors are treated separately, in the third section. Persons with low incomes have higher rates of disability caused by chronic conditions, but the differences are not as great as they are for the under-65 population and tend to fade as age increases and disability becomes more widespread. At age 85-plus, noninstitutionalized persons of low income appear to have less disability than higher-income persons, but that is undoubtedly misleading. At that age many disabled low-income persons will either be institutionalized and hence not counted or, because income is measured by families, will have shifted into a higher-income category because they have moved in with relatives who have income. Higher-income disabled persons by comparison are financially more able to maintain themselves in their own homes and to avoid or delay institutionalization.

The findings on race are consistent with those on income. Older nonwhites of all ages have more disability than whites. Part of the difference is a reflection of the higher income of whites. Presumably, cultural and other nonincome factors also have some effect. Elderly persons living in the South are somewhat more likely to report disabilities than their counterparts in other regions. Much of this difference is attributable to lower incomes in the South. Comparing rural with urban residents shows that elderly persons living in small towns and less populated areas are more apt to report chronic disabilities. These findings indicate that special efforts may be required to ensure that long-term-care programs reach those potentially most in need, particularly the poor and minority elderly.

In the third section we examine marital status and living arrangements as risk factors, factors which of course are greatly influenced by the difference in life expectancy between males and females. Combined data for noninstitutional and institutional populations confirm the findings from other research. Marital status and living arrangements are highly significant in determining who is at risk of being institutionalized or requiring long-term care provided from outside the immediate living arrangement. The survey data also indicate that these social factors are, at all ages over 65, at least as important as health factors in assessing the population at risk. Very large numbers of people who are unable to carry on their major activity because of serious chronic health conditions, including many in the 85-plus category, are able to remain in the community because they receive informal care and support from their relatives and friends. They become vulnerable to institutionalization not so much from a change in health status as from changes in marital status and living arrangement. If our goal is to prevent or delay institutionalization of the chronically ill elderly, these data suggest that we should focus as much effort on programs that encourage informal care and support as we now focus on those providing medical care.

In the final section we take a critical look at the current mix of medical and social programs for the elderly. The balance in federal spending on the over-65 population is steadily tilting toward medical spending and away from spending for other social purposes. The importance of living arrangements and other social factors suggests that this shift in policy is unfortunate. In our view, programs to bring elderly persons together with others in supportive social situations are likely to be more effective than policies designed to give them additional medical care.

Regardless of the relative importance of medical care, there are at least three aspects of the Medicare program that make it relatively inappropriate to a population where chronic illness is the prevalent health problem. First, Medicare coverage emphasizes episodic acute hospital care, whereas the illnesses affecting the elderly, by their nature, require continuous management, ideally outside of hospitals. Second, insurance plans such as Medicare are financial devices, not programs for reaching out to identify the chronically ill and guiding them toward ongoing appropriate care. The result is that many elderly end up with inadequate or unnecessary care. Finally, the traditional fee-for-service, cost reimbursement method of payment, which Medicare uses, results in distorted incentives. Rather than rewarding health professionals for the proper management of chronic illness and the prevention of acute flare-ups requiring hospitalization, it can actually reward mismanagement by paying for the resulting more costly care.

The Health Status of Older Persons

For the purposes of public policy, measurement of health status is essential to determining the need for health resources and services. Several studies suggest that the definition and measurement of the health of older persons should focus on functional ability rather than the presence or absence of disease (Haber 1967; Shanas 1971; Lawton 1971; Maddox 1964). This is largely due to evidence that though many older persons suffer from chronic disease or impairment of some kind, the impact of such conditions varies widely within the population (Shanas 1962, 1971; Kovar 1977). Therefore, although functional ability is an indirect measure of health, it provides a better picture of the health resources and services an aged person will require (Shanas and Maddox 1976; World Health Organization 1959). Moreover, Maddox and Douglass (1973) found that when compared with medical diagnoses, functional self assessments were better predictors of health status over time.

In this study we use functional ability as determined through interviews conducted by the national Health Interview Survey (HIS).[2] Each year, this survey gathers information on the health of about 110,000 persons who are a representative sample of the U.S. civilian population not living in institutions. About 10 percent of those persons are over 65 years old. The analysis here is based largely on unpublished data from the 1976 and 1977 surveys and provides a picture of the health of older persons in three age groups—65 through 74; 75 through 84; and 85 and over. In examining the health status of those groups in this section we use two broad functional measures, daily health status and chronic disability, and list the leading chronic conditions which cause both those measures to decline with age. Unless otherwise noted, all data presented in this and the following section examine separately survey data for the population residing in institutions.

Daily Health Status across Age

The HIS measures daily health status by restricted activity days and bed disability days. Restricted activity days, which are the broadest measure of disability collected by the survey, can result from chronic or acute conditions and include days spent in bed, days lost from work or school, and any day when an individual decreases his or her normal activities for the whole day. Bed disability days, a component of restricted activity days, are days when most or all of the day is spent in bed because of illness or injury (NCHS 1978).

In figure 2.1 data are presented on the annual number of restricted activity days, including bed disability days, per person by age group. As expected, the data show that younger age groups report many fewer re-

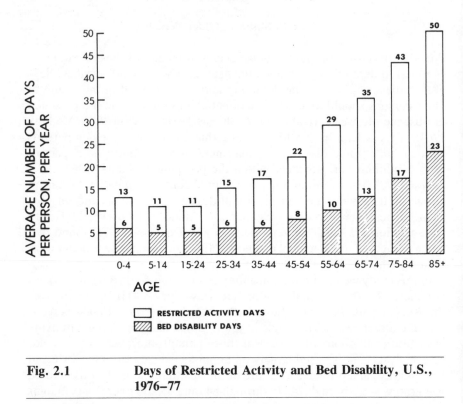

AVERAGE NUMBER OF DAYS PER PERSON, PER YEAR

AGE

☐ RESTRICTED ACTIVITY DAYS
▨ BED DISABILITY DAYS

Fig. 2.1   **Days of Restricted Activity and Bed Disability, U.S., 1976–77**

stricted activity days than do older age groups. The only exception is the very young. Between the 0–4 group and 5–14 group there is a decline in the number of restricted activity days per person. This trend reverses with the 15–24 group. At this point, restricted activity days begin to rise as age increases. The rise is continuous and not abrupt. Thus, the greater number days of restricted activity among the elderly are the result of a trend that begins at an early age and not a phenomenon that appears suddenly in later years. Even after age 65, the rate of increase remains fairly stable.

Restricted activity days are associated with either acute or chronic conditions. Figure 2.2 shows that acute conditions account for a high proportion of restricted activity days among the young and chronic conditions for a high proportion among the old. A steady shift is evident across age: as age increases, chronic conditions account for a greater proportion of restricted activity.

The most striking aspect of the data on restricted activity days is, as figure 2.2 shows, that days of restricted activity due to acute conditions are similar for all ages. For example, of an average of about 50 restricted

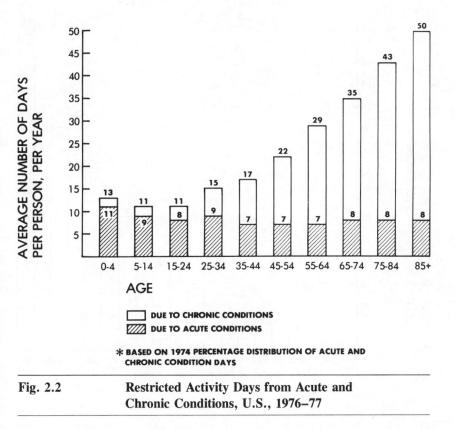

**Fig. 2.2   Restricted Activity Days from Acute and
Chronic Conditions, U.S., 1976–77**

days a year for persons 85 and over, only 8 of those days are attributable
to acute illness. The only age groups with a lower number of such days are
those from 35 to 64, and they average about 7 days a year. The higher
level of restricted activity reported by the elderly is then attributable
entirely to chronic conditions, including acute episodes attributable to
those conditions.

Chronic Disability

Showing that chronic illnesses account for most of the day-to-day illness
among the elderly does not tell us how many of the aged may need long-
term care. Such day-to-day illness may be spread evenly across the elderly
population or concentrated among relatively few people. The "limitation
of activity" classification of the Health Interview Survey offers a way of
determining the degree to which health problems associated with chronic
illness are concentrated among the elderly.

Each year interviewers ask people whether they are limited in activity

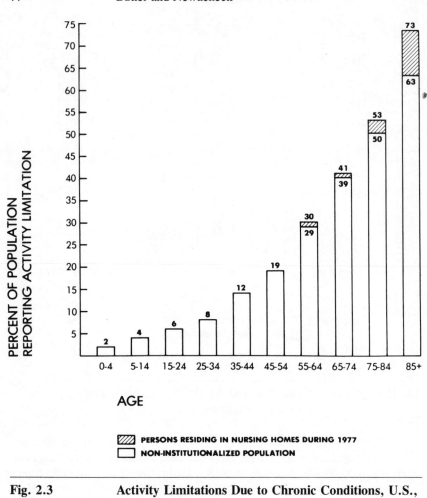

PERCENT OF POPULATION REPORTING ACTIVITY LIMITATION

AGE

▨ PERSONS RESIDING IN NURSING HOMES DURING 1977
☐ NON-INSTITUTIONALIZED POPULATION

Fig. 2.3   **Activity Limitations Due to Chronic Conditions, U.S., 1976–77**

because of chronic health problems. Based on the questionnaire responses people are classified in one of four categories: (1) not limited in activity; (2) limited, but not in their major activity, as a result of chronic conditions; (3) limited in the kind or amount of major activity, as a result of chronic conditions, or; (4) unable to carry on their major activity, as a result of chronic conditions. Major activity refers to work for adult males, housework or work for adult females, and play or school attendance for children.[3]

The prevalence of chronic limitation of activity naturally increases with age and at an increasing rate. But, contrary to popular perception, the increase is steady, consistent with the steady increase in days of restricted

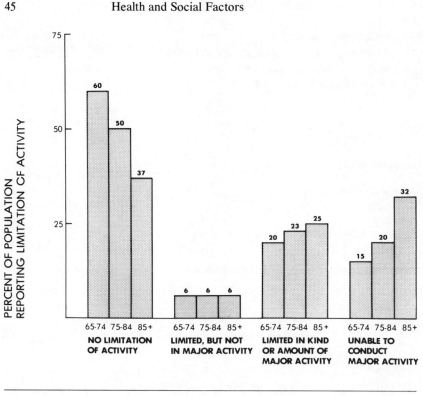

Fig. 2.4   Activity Limitation Due to Chronic Conditions, U.S., 1976–77

activity shown in figure 2.1. Figure 2.3 shows the proportion of each age group reporting some degree of limitation of activity due to chronic conditions. The proportion reporting such limitations rises from about 2 percent among the youngest children (0–4 years) to 63 percent for the oldest group (85+ years). Although persons 65 and over report limitations of activity due to chronic conditions about five times as frequently as those under 65, the increase in prevalence is not abrupt at any point. If one assumes that persons residing in nursing homes are also limited in activity, the curve would look steeper for the total population. When data on the nursing home population are added as indicated by the shaded areas in figure 2.3, the curve still shows a relatively steady increase, but with a larger jump at age 85+, where a relatively large proportion of the population lives in nursing homes.

HIS classifies people with impaired ability to carry on their activities as either "unable to conduct major activity," or "limited in amount or kind of major activity," or "limited, but not in major activity." Figure 2.4 shows how the severity of disability increases with age among the elderly.

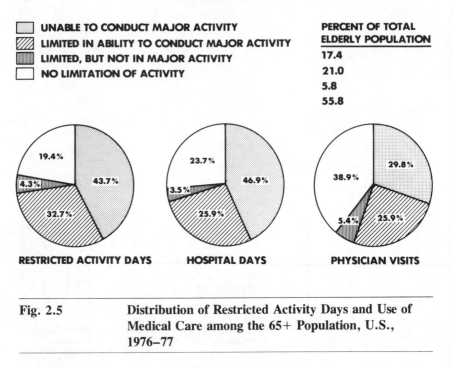

Fig. 2.5   **Distribution of Restricted Activity Days and Use of Medical Care among the 65+ Population, U.S., 1976–77**

The percentage of persons unable to carry on their major activity shows the greatest increase. In contrast, the percentage "limited, but not in major activity" increases only slightly.

Although disability becomes more severe with age, figure 2.4 shows that it is confined to a relatively small percentage of the elderly. For example, only 20 percent of the 75 to 84 age group are unable to carry on their major activity, and half of the people in this age group do not report any disability. Even at ages 85+ the percentage with no disability of any kind is higher than the percentage unable to carry on their major activity.

These data show that disability is concentrated in a limited group of the elderly. When disability is related to days of restricted activity among the elderly and their use of medical care, the concentration is equally apparent. Figure 2.5 shows that the 17 percent of the elderly who are unable to carry on their major activity account for 44 percent of the restricted activity days and 47 percent of hospital days. In rough terms, approximately one-fifth of those over 65 account for half of the health problems. The proportion of physician visits accounted for by the severely disabled is markedly lower (30 percent) because the less disabled and more ambulatory elderly are relatively high users of physicians.

The amount of daily illness and hospital use among the elderly seems to depend entirely on the degree of disability. Figures 2.6 and 2.7 show that

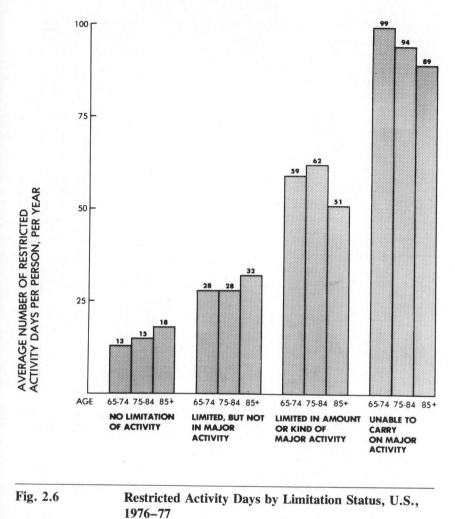

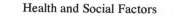

Fig. 2.6   **Restricted Activity Days by Limitation Status, U.S.,
1976–77**

---

it is level of disability, rather than age, that accounts for the substantial
differences in the number of restricted activity and hospital days reported
by the elderly. That is, when the elderly are divided into activity limitation
categories, there are only minor differences in daily health and hospital
use across age.

The impact of limitation of activity on restricted activity days is clear
from figure 2.6. Elderly persons without limitation of activity report from
13 (age 65–74) to 18 (age 85+) days of restricted activity annually, similar
to the 16 days reported by the U.S. population under 65. Those with
activity limitation but not in their major activity report about twice the

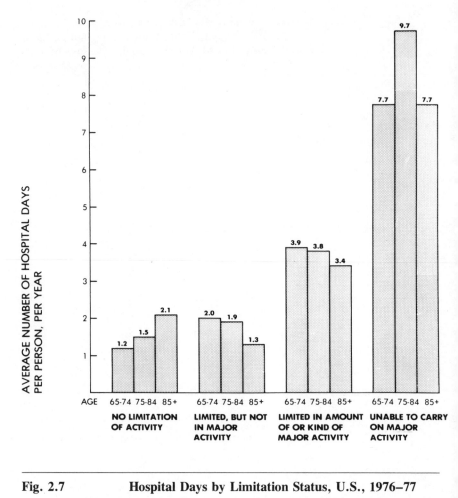

Fig. 2.7   **Hospital Days by Limitation Status, U.S., 1976–77**

number of days as those without limitation; those limited in the amount or kind of major activity report about three times that number; and those with the most severe form of limitation report almost 100 restricted activity days annually, or about 2 days per week—five times the rate of those without limitations. The same pattern holds for hospital use, illustrated in figure 2.7. For example, those who are unable to conduct their major activity spend about four to five times the number of days in the hospital and report about twice the number of physician visits as those without limitation, whose rates of utilization are similar to the under-65 population.

Table 2.1	The 10 Leading Chronic Conditions Reported as Main Cause of Limitation of Activity among Persons 65 and Over, U.S., 1977
Chronic Condition	**Percent of elderly limited by chronic condition**
1. Heart disease	8.0
2. Arthritis and chronic rheumatism	7.6
3. Senility	3.0
4. Impairments, lower extremities and hips	2.0
5. Hypertensive disease	2.0
6. Emphysema	1.7
7. Arteriosclerosis and other chronic disease of the circulatory system	1.5
8. Cerebrovascular disease	1.4
9. Impairments, back and spine	1.2
10. Diabetes (mellitus)	1.2

Leading Chronic Conditions

Heart disease, arthritis, and chronic rheumatism have a much greater impact on the aged than other chronic conditons (see table 2.1). The number of elderly limited in activity due to heart disease is greater than the total number limited in activity due to hypertension, emphysema, cerebrovascular disease, impairments of the back and spine, and diabetes. The prevalence of all major chronic conditions increases with age but at markedly different rates depending on the condition. The increase is more abrupt for conditions with a later onset, such as heart conditions, arthritis, and rheumatism, which are rare in persons under 30. It is quite gradual for hypertension and impairments of lower extremities and hips, which appear earlier in life but whose progress is slow, although steady. Senility is the only major chronic condition that appears only in the 65 and over age group.

Relevance of Some Socioeconomic and Demographic Factors

In this section we analyze the relationships between several demographic and socioeconomic variables and prevalence of limitation of major activity among the elderly. Persons limited in major activity include individuals who are limited in the amount or kind of their major activity and those who are unable to carry on their major activity. Again in this section, unless otherwise noted the data presented refer to the noninstitutional population.

Sex

In 1977, the aged population was composed of three-fifths females and two-fifths males. Largely because of different mortality rates, women account for much larger proportions of the "old-old" than they do of the "young-old." As table 2.2 shows for the noninstitutionalized population, there are about 1.3 females for each male between the ages of 65 and 75, but after age 85 women outnumber men by more than 2 to 1.

Table 2.2	Sex Distribution of Elderly Noninstitutional Population		
65+	**65–74**	**75–84**	**85+**
males			
41%	43%	38%	32%
females			
59%	57%	62%	68%

Women do not dominate the disabled population to the degree that they dominate the elderly population generally (see table 2.3). Although there are greater numbers of women limited in their major activity than men, prevalence of such limitation is greater among men. Overall, 44 percent of elderly males (4.0 million) were limited in major activity compared with 35 percent of the women (4.5 million) during 1976–77. The differences in prevalence are greatest among the younger elderly and diminish with increased age. By age 85 disability levels are nearly equal, with about three-fifths of each sex reporting chronic disabilities.

The difference in prevalence of disability between sexes may be attributable to a number of factors. Elderly men have been exposed to a greater number of risk factors, particularly occupational, than have women. Men also have shorter life spans than women. For example, average life expectancy at age 65 is currently about 5 years less for males. Finally, elderly women reside in nursing homes at nearly twice the rate as males, leaving a more healthy female noninstitutional population.

Table 2.3	Persons Limited in Major Activity, by Sex		
65+	65–74	75–84	85+
males 44%	40%	50%	59%
females 35%	30%	39%	57%

For the most part these factors diminish in importance with advanced age, leading to a more equalized distribution of disability between the sexes by age 85. While institutionalization rates are still higher for females, past exposure to occupational risk factors becomes less important in predicting current limitations. Life expectancy differences are also reduced. At age 85, life expectancy differs by only about one year between the sexes. Hence, the overall narrowing of disability of differences.

The data do reveal another difference between males and females. At all ages over 65, proportionately more males than females are unable to carry on their major activity. Thirty percent of elderly males report such limitations compared with 9 percent of females. Conversely, more females are limited in the kind or amount of their major activity, with 26 percent of aged females and 14 percent aged males reporting this level of disability. These differences do, however, narrow as age increases.

Other researchers have speculated that much of this difference is accounted for by the nature of questions asked in the Health Interview Survey (Shanas and Maddox 1976). The major activity of an older male is defined to be work in the sense of labor force participation. Women, in contrast, are also asked about housekeeping and are therefore more apt to report that they are limited in their ability to carry out their major activity rather than totally unable to do so. In any event the difference seems insignificant for policy purposes.

Income

Although income levels among the elderly have increased substantially over the past two decades, 40 percent of those over 65 (7.4 million) reported family income levels below $5,000 during 1976–77. It is also apparent from table 2.4 that income diminishes with age. Between the ages of 65–74 and 85+, there is a 47 percent increase in the proportion of elderly with family incomes falling below $5,000. This loss of income occurs for a number of reasons, including eroded value of pension income due to the effects of inflation, declining asset income, and in part, reduced family income through the loss of a spouse.

Table 2.4	Income Distribution of Elderly Noninstitutional Population		
65+	65–74	75–84	85+
Family income less than $5000			
39%	34%	47%	50%
Family income $5000 or more			
61%	66%	53%	50%

Note: Excludes persons with unknown income; income from all sources is included, e.g., wages, rents, pensions, and help from relatives.

We would expect that older persons of low income would be less healthy than other elderly, and this is the case. When the percentage distribution of disability by income is examined, it shows that the under $5,000 income group has a disproportionately higher share of disability. Low income seems to have two effects, both visible in these data. It leads to lower levels of nutrition, housing, health care, and other necessities and therefore to greater likelihood that a chronic health condition will develop or become worse. The results of this effect are evident in the 65 to 84 age group, where disability is more prevalent among the poor (see table 2.5).

Table 2.5	Percent of Persons Limited in Major Activity, by Income		
65+	65–74	75–84	85+
Family income less than $5000			
46%	44%	48%	55%
Family income $5000 or more			
35%	30%	41%	61%

As age progresses and disabilities become more common, income has another effect. Higher income increases ability to purchase in-home assistance and care, thus reducing the likelihood of institutionalization. On the other hand, lack of necessary financial resources to remain in the community on the part of those with low incomes and severe disabilities increases their likelihood of being institutionalized (Berg, et al., 1970; Dunlop 1975; Davis and Gibbon 1971).

This effect begins to appear in the over-75 population, and becomes very visible in the 85 and over segment of the group. Noninstitutionalized low-income persons 85 and over actually report less disability than their higher-income counterparts. A possible explanation for this result, then, is that a higher percentage of the low-income disabled group are institutionalized because they lack financial resources, while proportionately

Table 2.6	Race Distribution of Elderly Noninstitutional Population		
65+	**65–74**	**75–84**	**85+**
white			
91%	90%	91%	90%
nonwhite			
9%	10%	9%	10%

more disabled persons with higher incomes are able to remain in the community. In addition, the higher rates of disability among higher-income elderly are due to the method by which income is measured. That is, as older low-income disabled people move in with family members, they assume a higher-income status because income is measured by family units in the survey.

Race

Nonwhites accounted for 9.4 percent (2.1 million) of the noninstitutionalized elderly population during 1976–77, substantially less than the population generally (13.4 percent during 1977) (see table 2.6). The under-

Table 2.7	Persons Limited in Major Activity, by Race		
65+	**65–74**	**75–84**	**85+**
white			
37%	33%	43%	56%
nonwhite			
47%	43%	52%	68%

representation of nonwhites among the elderly is due to a number of factors including differences in longevity by race.

Since life expectancy at birth is lower for nonwhites than for whites, we might expect to see a declining share of nonwhites as age increases. Table 2.6 indicates that this is not the case. The reasons for this circumstance are twofold: nonwhites have similar life expectancies as whites by age 60 or 65, and elderly nonwhites are less likely to reside in nursing homes. (Scanlon 1978)

At all ages in the U.S. population, nonwhites exhibit greater levels of disability than do whites. Table 2.7 shows that 47 percent of elderly nonwhites reported being limited in major activity during 1976–77, compared with only 37 percent of whites. Nonwhites in each age group are more likely to report disabilities.

Table 2.8	Regional Distribution of Elderly Noninstitutional Population		
65+	65–74	75–84	85+
Northeast 24%	23%	25%	23%
North Central 27%	27%	28%	27%
South 33%	33%	32%	33%
West 16%	17%	16%	18%

Region

The aged population is distributed across the U.S. in a similar fashion to the general population (see table 2.8). More elderly people live in the South than in any other region of the country. The West is the smallest region in terms of its over-65 population, with only half of that of the South.

For a number of reasons we would expect greater levels of disability in the South compared with other regions. First, the South is more rural—36 percent of those living in the South live in nonmetropolitan areas, as compared with 22 percent in the three other regions. Second, incomes are

Table 2.9	Persons Limited in Major Activity, by Region		
65+	65–74	75–84	85+
Northeast 34%	30%	38%	56%
North Central 36%	33%	40%	50%
South 43%	38%	51%	62%
West 39%	34%	43%	61%

lower in the South—45 percent of the elderly living in the South had family incomes of less that $5,000 during 1976–77 as compared with 36 percent in the other regions.

Institutionalization rates differ by region as well, and should have an effect on the disability levels reported by the noninstitutional population. Rates of institutionalization are substantially lower in the South as compared with the three other regions. Scanlon (1978) suggests that much of these differences are due to lower Medicaid reimbursement levels in the

South. Another factor affecting institutionalization rates is climatic differences. Scanlon found that, after controlling for a number of variables, utilization of nursing homes is 30 to 40 percent greater in states in the northern plains or upper Midwest as compared with the Deep South because of harsher winters in the former. Because of these differences in institutionalization and other factors, higher rates of disability would be expected among the noninstitutionalized elderly in the South when compared with other regions.

Data presented in table 2.9 indicate that such expected differences do in fact exist. Compared with the other regions, aged persons living in the South are about 20 percent more likely to report a chronic condition resulting in limitation of major activity than are their counterparts in the remainder of the U.S. Although not shown, almost all of this excessive prevalence is in the form of the most severe disability—inability to conduct one's major activity. These differences tend to narrow with increased age, but they are substantial enough to warrant increased policy attention to the long-term-care needs of the South.

Residence

In 1977 approximately 37 percent of the noninstitutionalized aged lived in nonmetropolitan areas as compared with 32 percent for the entire U.S., suggesting that the problems of aging are of particular significance to small towns and rural areas.

Table 2.10	Residence Distribution of Elderly Noninstitutional Population		
65+	65–74	75–84	85+
SMSA			
63%	63%	63%	62%
Non-SMSA			
37%	37%	37%	38%

Also, rural areas, particularly in the South, have historically reported higher levels of acute and chronic illness, inadequate medical resources, lower incomes, and environmental and occupational hazards. While studies on nursing home institutionalization rates show no consistent differences between the urban and rural elderly (Davis and Gibbon 1971; Scanlon 1978), the high proportion of rural elderly living in the South (where institutionalization rates have been shown to be low) might result in higher rates of disability among the noninstitutionalized rural aged.

The data in table 2.11 indicate that differences in disability levels do exist but these differences narrow with increasing age.

Table 2.11	Persons Limited in Major Activity, by Residence		
65+	65–74	75–84	85+
SMSA 36%	32%	41%	57%
Non-SMSA 42%	38%	47%	58%

Marital Status and Living Arrangements

In a large study of nursing home admission patterns in western New York State, Davis and Gibbon found that, regardless of functional status, elderly persons admitted to nursing homes tended to be unmarried, over 75, and female, whereas those remaining in the community tended to possess the opposite characteristics (David and Gibbon 1971). The authors conclude that "marital status, age, and sex are apparently better predictors of the likelihood of nursing home placement than functional characteristics" (p. 1150). Other studies carried out in the United States and England have shown that between 5 and 20 percent of the elderly admitted to institutions were admitted primarily for social reasons (NCHS 1977b; Haberstein and Biddle 1974; Brockington and Lempert 1966). Dunlop (1974), in summarizing the available evidence, asserts that "the medical conditions of most elderly admittees to nursing home type facilities are shared by many other elderly persons residing in the community, but the social situations [broadly defined by Dunlop to include financial status] of the admittees are different; and it is this, it seems, which often accounts for their admission" (p. 14).

The biggest source of support for disabled persons in the community is a husband or wife. Without such support the older person is particularly vulnerable. Both the 1970 census and the 1973–74 Nursing Home Survey indicate that the institutionalized elderly include three times as high a proportion of never-married persons as are found in the community. Similarly, the nursing home population contains almost twice the proportion of widows as would be expected based on the proportion in the noninstitutional elderly population. Shanas (1979), commenting on those relationships, suggests: "These findings are what one would expect. Persons without close family ties are more likely to be institutionalized when they are old.... Old persons with few or limited family relationships are prime candidates for institutionalization when they become sick" (p. 171).

This section assesses the importance of marital status and living arrangements in delaying institutionalization. We start by looking at trends in marital status among the aged to see how many of the elderly are widowed and at what ages. Then trends in living arrangement across age and sex are examined to determine what happens to those elderly who are widowed and how that varies with their health status. Finally, we compare the distribution of the noninstitutionalized population by marital status, living arrangement, sex, and age with that of the nursing home population to learn how marital status and living arrangements affect utilization of nursing homes.

Trends in Marital Status and Living Arrangements

Overall, half of the elderly not living in institutions are married, two-fifths are widowed, and one-tenth are in the category of divorced, separated, or never married. Although the proportions of divorced, separated, or never-married persons is constant across age, there are very visible trends in the proportions of married and widowed persons. The most important trend is the loss of a spouse. Between the ages of 65 and 74, some 3.5 million people are widowed, accounting for more than a fourth of all persons in that age group. With increasing age, the number of widows and widowers quickly exceeds the number of married. By age 85, there are three and one-half times as many widowed as married persons (see table 2.12).

The loss of a spouse after years of companionship is not only traumatic in itself but is usually accompanied by two drastic changes in life style. First, income is often reduced. Among the elderly, widowed persons are twice as likely to fall below the poverty line as are married persons. Second, the aged person without a spouse may quickly become socially isolated unless old bonds are strengthened or new relationships are initiated.

Most who are widowed live alone. Sixty percent (4.5 million) of the widowed elderly live alone through choice or lack of alternatives. The remaining 3 million live, for the most part, with other relatives and less often with nonrelatives. With increasing age and reduced health status, fewer of those widowed live alone. After age 85, a majority live with others compared with 36 percent of those aged 65–74 and 40 percent of those aged 75–84. In each age group only about 10 percent of those living with others live with nonrelatives. This supports Shanas's findings (1979) that older people first turn to their children in time of need, then to other relatives if children are unavailable, and finally to friends and neighbors.

While nearly 2 million widows and widowers aged 75 and older live alone, many have substantial social contacts. Shanas (1968) in a 1962–63 survey found that about 75 percent of widowed elderly living alone had

Table 2.12	Marital Status and Living Arrangements of the Noninstitutional Population, U.S., 1973–74	

Both Sexes

65–74	Population Distribution (by percent)	Percent Limited in Major Activity
Married	62.3	34.0
Widowed	27.3	34.3
Alone	63.9	31.6
Relatives	33.0	38.8
Nonrelatives	3.0	42.0
Never married/ Div/Sep	10.4	35.9
Alone	56.7	35.5
Relatives	35.7	36.4
Nonrelatives	7.6	36.6
	100%	

75–84		
Married	42.1	45.7
Widowed	48.6	42.7
Alone	60.5	35.4
Relatives	36.1	54.3
Nonrelatives	3.4	48.9
Never married/ Div/Sep	9.3	38.7
Alone	53.9	36.1
Relatives	38.0	40.9
Nonrelatives	8.1	45.9*
	100%	

85+		
Married	20.5	58.1
Widowed	70.5	57.0
Alone	43.0	48.0
Relatives	52.4	64.5
Nonrelatives	4.6	55.8*
Never married/ Div/Sep	9.0	59.1
Alone	48.9	55.6
Relatives	39.3	63.4
Nonrelatives	11.9*	59.7*
	100%	

*Figure does not meet NCHS standards of reliability or precision (see appendix).

seen a child in the week prior to the interview. However, 25 percent either had no children or had not seen a child in the previous week. This latter group was also the most likely to report being "lonely" in the interviews.

Those who are divorced, separated, or never married (mostly the latter) account for about 10 percent of the noninstitutional population in each elderly age group. In comparison with widowed persons, we would expect fewer close family ties in this group and greater proportions living alone. However, up until age 85 this is not the case. Between 65 and 85 more of this group live with others than is the case with widows and widowers. In fact, a greater proportion of those between 65 and 85 lives with relatives than widowed persons in the same age group. After age 85 the situation is reversed and proportionately more widowed persons live with relatives, probably because relatively few of the divorced, separated, or never-married elderly have children. That is, relatives for this group probably tend to be brothers and sisters, and by age 85 many of these are deceased or institutionalized themselves. In each age group these unmarried persons are two or more times as likely to live with nonrelatives as are widowed persons.

Differences by Sex

While the proportions of persons divorced, separated, or never married not living in institutions are almost equal by sex, the proportions of married and widowed differ greatly. Only about one-third of elderly women are married as compared with three-fourths of men, largely because women live longer and usually have older husbands. Tables 2.13 and 2.14 show that at age 65–74 men are almost twice as likely to be married but at age 85 and after are more than five times as likely to be married. At that age there are 10 widowed women for each married woman, while the numbers of widowed and married men are roughly equal. It is largely these differences in marital status that account for the disproportionate number of women in nursing homes.

There are no major differences in the living arrangements of widows and widowers. Both predominately tend to live alone, until very old age (85+). Males are slightly more likely to live with nonrelatives than are females, but about equally likely to live with relatives. Among the divorced, separated, or never married, we see the same general trends: the majority of each sex lives alone until 85 or so, and both sexes depend on relatives more than on friends.

Differences by Disability

There is little difference in disability by marital status (table 2.12). Larger differences are visible in living arrangements. Because of the difficulties

Table 2.13	Limitation Status of the Male Noninstitutional Population, U.S., 1973–74	
65–74	**Population Distribution (by percent)**	**Percent Limited in Major Activity**
Married	80.7	38.8
Widowed	9.6	42.4
Alone	60.2	39.3
Relatives	35.4	45.3
Nonrelatives	4.5*	61.3*
Never married/ Div/Sep	9.7	42.4
Alone	56.8	43.4
Relatives	33.7	40.7
Nonrelatives	9.5	42.2*
	100%	
75–84		
Married	68.8	49.6
Widowed	22.7	48.4
Alone	56.2	42.2
Relatives	39.3	57.5
Nonrelatives	4.6*	47.4*
Never married/ Div/Sep	8.6	47.8
Alone	52.5	45.3
Relatives	37.9	51.9
Nonrelatives	9.6*	45.6*
	100%	
85+		
Married	44.7	59.5
Widowed	47.7	59.7
Alone	44.6	54.6
Relatives	52.7	63.7
Nonrelatives	2.7*	64.3*
Never married/ Div/Sep	7.6	76.2*
Alone	48.7*	78.3*
Relatives	35.9*	77.9*
Nonrelatives	15.4*	65.6*
	100%	

*Figure does not meet NCHS standards of reliability or precision (see appendix).

Table 2.14   **Limitation Status of the Female Noninstitutional Population, U.S., 1973–74**

65–74	Population Distribution (by percent)	Percent Limited in Major Activity
Married	48.3	27.7
Widowed	40.8	32.9
Alone	64.6	30.4
Relatives	32.6	37.5
Nonrelatives	2.8	36.3
Never married/ Div/Sep	10.9	31.5
Alone	56.5	30.1
Relatives	37.1	33.8
Nonrelatives	6.3	30.8*
	100%	

75–84		
Married	25.2	38.9
Widowed	65.0	41.4
Alone	61.5	34.0
Relatives	35.4	53.5
Nonrelatives	3.1	49.4
Never married/ Div/Sep	9.8	33.7
Alone	54.7	31.2
Relatives	38.1	34.8
Nonrelatives	7.3	46.2*
	100%	

85+		
Married	8.0	54.3
Widowed	82.3	56.2
Alone	42.5	45.9
Relatives	52.3	64.8
Nonrelatives	5.2	54.5*
Never married/ Div/Sep	9.7	52.2
Alone	48.9	46.4*
Relatives	40.6	58.2
Nonrelatives	10.5*	56.2*
	100%	

*Figure does not meet NCHS standards of reliability or precision (see appendix).

of living alone with a disability, we would expect more of the disabled elderly to live with others, and they do. For example between the ages of 75 and 84, 54 percent of widowed persons living with relatives are limited in major activity, as compared with 35 percent of widows and widowers living alone (table 2.12). Similar patterns also are seen in the divorced, separated, or never-married elderly, although these patterns are somewhat less apparent than for the widowed.

The picture that emerges, then, is of the disabled unmarried elderly turning to relatives and friends for assistance in carrying out their usual activities. However, there are still nearly 2 million aged persons living alone with limitations in major activity, a group that is highly vulnerable.

Effect on Institutionalization

By using another source of data on the elderly nursing home population, the risk of institutionalization for unmarried persons, particularly those living alone, can be seen. This is done by comparing rates of nursing home institutionalization by marital status and living arrangement. Rates of institutionalization are calculated across age, marital status, living arrangement, and sex in table 2.15 by dividing the nursing home population by the combined total of the noninstitutional and nursing home population for each combination of variables.

These rates are based on data from the 1973–74 National Nursing Home Survey (NNHS) and the Health Interview Survey from the same years. The NNHS focused on nursing homes and personal-care-with-nursing homes. Since only two-fifths of the nursing home population were admitted directly from private residences, living arrangements were estimated for the other three-fifths who were admittedly indirectly (in most cases from hospitals or other institutions). Living arrangements prior to institutionalization for those admitted indirectly were estimated by assuming that their living arrangements were identical to those admitted directly in each sex, age, and marital status category. Also, since the nursing home survey asked about current marital status, some of the elderly in nursing homes who are currently widowed may have been married at the time of admission. However, this error is likely to be a small one since less than 10 percent of the currently widowed lived with a spouse prior to admission. The lack of perfect information suggests caution, however, in interpreting small differences in estimates of institutionalization rates.

The first column of table 2.15 shows rates of nursing home institutionalization by marital status for both sexes combined. Because of substantial social support provided by a spouse, we would expect lower rates for the married elderly in each group, and that is the case. Widows and widowers are up to five times more likely to be institutionalized than are

Table 2.15   Estimated Institutionalization Rates, U.S., 1973–74

Percent of Population Residing in Nursing Homes

	Both Sexes	Males	Females
65–74			
Married	.4	.3	.4
Widowed	2.1	3.2	1.9
Alone	1.3	2.1	1.2
Relatives	3.4	4.4	3.2
Nonrelatives	3.9*	6.9*	3.0*
Never married/			
Div/Sep	4.1	5.5	3.1
Alone	2.6	4.0	1.8
Relatives	6.5	8.8	4.9
Nonrelatives	3.8*	2.1*	4.7*
75–84			
Married	2.0	1.7	2.6
Widowed	7.9	7.8	7.9
Alone	5.6	6.2	5.5
Relatives	11.6	10.3	11.9
Nonrelatives	7.6	5.3	8.3
Never married/			
Div/Sep	10.2	11.4	9.5
Alone	10.0	11.9	9.1
Relatives	11.1	12.4	10.3
Nonrelatives	7.0*	4.3*	8.6*
85+			
Married	11.3	9.2	17.0
Widowed	27.5	24.3	28.4
Alone	26.1	22.4	27.1
Relatives	29.3	26.2	30.2
Nonrelatives	18.1	18.5*	18.1
Never married/			
Div/Sep	32.3	32.1	32.3
Alone	35.9	32.0*	36.8
Relatives	30.6	34.1*	29.2
Nonrelatives	21.1*	25.8*	18.8*

Note: Estimates based on data from the 1973–74 National Nursing Home Survey and the 1973–74 Health Interview Survey (see appendix for actual computations).

*Figure does not meet NCHS standards of reliability or precision (see appendix).

married persons. Further, those least likely to have available and able relatives to care for them—the divorced, separated, or never married—have up to ten times the rate of institutionalization of married persons. In each case these differences appear not to be explained by differences in the prevalence of limitation of major activity, since such differences are quite small (see table 2.12). Thus, a person's social situation has a substantial effect on whether he or she ends up in a nursing home.

These marital differences in institutionalization are evident for each sex. In fact, the disproportionate number of women in nursing homes is largely explained when men are compared with women by age and marital status. For each age group rates of institutionalization for unmarried men and women are almost equal. That is, more women are in nursing homes, not because they are less healthy, but because they are older and more likely to be unmarried.

The only consistent difference in nursing home admissions by sex is for the married elderly. In each age group, married males are less likely to be institutionalized than married women. This difference is most likely due to different ages between spouses. Women are likely to have older and less able spouses to care for them. The reverse is more often the case for men.

The difficulty that older spouses have in caring for one another also appears to account for the declining edge that married people have over the unmarried with increasing age, a trend observable in table 2.15. At age 65 to 74 the unmarried are about six times more likely to be institutionalized than are the married. By age 85 the ratio is reduced to about two to one.

Among the unmarried elderly, we would expect differences in living arrangement to affect the likelihood of nursing home placement. Those living with others should have higher rates of institutionalization because they are more often disabled, which is frequently their reasons for moving in with others. Table 2.15 shows that this is the case. Further, since disability levels are lowest for the unmarried living alone as compared with all other living arrangements, based on health factors this group should have the lowest institutionalization rate. They do have lower rates than unmarrieds living with other relatives, but they have much higher rates than the married elderly who are less healthy but have a spouse to care for them. The difference is the vulnerability of those living alone with a disability.

Living alone, relative to living with others, also becomes more risky with age. Between 65 and 74 those who are unmarried and living alone are substantially less likely to be institutionalized than those who are unmarried but living with others. By age 85, living alone results in an equal or greater chance of institutionalization as compared with living with relatives or nonrelatives, even though those living alone are on average healthier.

Discussion of Social Support Alternatives

Despite the fact that most of those living alone can depend on their families to take care of them in time of need, a substantial minority lack such assurances. In a three-generation family study, Litman (1971) found that while about 80 percent of the families expressed the view that convalescent care at home is most desirable, about one-third said they would not provide such care under any circumstances. Similarly, a study in Massachusetts found that while 70 percent of families were willing to take care of an elderly family member after a first hospitalization, only 38 percent would do so after a second hospital episode (Eggert, et al., 1977).

To make matters worse, those without family support are more likely to be poor. Some 31 percent of those living alone during 1975 had incomes below the poverty standard, while the figure was 15 percent for the elderly in general. The combination of isolation and low income can be devastating to a person's mental and physical health. Data from the Health Interview Survey show that those living alone with low incomes are more likely to report limitation of major activity than those with higher incomes. In fact, one and one-half million elderly persons were living alone with limitation of major activity and incomes of $400 or less per month ($5,000 per year) during 1976–77. Under such circumstances it is not surprising that institutionalization rates are high.

The absence of supportive family care may be the result of competing demands on family resources of time, energy, space, or money. Sussman (1976) suggests that families might be able and willing to provide more care for their elderly kin if various supports were provided to ease the burdens that such care imposes. He states that "one logical substitute for the continued proliferation of impersonal institutions and large bureaucratic agencies is the channeling of some of the funds used for service provision directly to the families of the elderly who can provide more personalized care at perhaps lower cost." Breslau and Haug (1972) concluded as a result of a demonstration project that "the needed social service would be more effective if it elicited the cooperation of the family and were perceived and formulated as a family enterprise. In other words, social service, instead of being an independent and alternative agent of intervention, ought to attempt to be a family ally that offers assistance when caring for the aged member is too great a burden." Sussman further suggests that although most elderly living with relatives live with one of their children, it is possible that other, more distant members of the family network, such as grandchildren, nephews, siblings, etc., would also be willing to undertake the care of elderly relatives if the added responsibility were offset by certain financial or service benefits.

Where family ties are absent or so tenuous as to preclude effective support networks, surrogate forms of family support are possible. Such forms include congregate facilities or boarding homes with groups of more self-sufficient elderly members assisting other groups of more functionally dependent older persons. Given the proper incentives and interest, the possibilities for such supportive networks are considerable, since 150,000 of the elderly are currently estimated to live in boardinghouses or other group quarters, and another 750,000 live in public housing, in which most units are age segregated (Carp 1976). Other forms of potentially supportive living include domiciliary care facilities, congregate housing, retirement communities, trailer parks, and sheltered housing.

Some living arrangements may be more effective than others in maintaining the physical and mental health of a particular older individual. It is important to remember that the elderly population is probably the most heterogeneous population of all (Kelly 1955). Physical, emotional, and psychological differences reach their peak in old age, so that one living situation, be it family, shared housing with a friend, or even living alone, may be most appropriate for one person but least appropriate for another. Carp (1976) suggests that little is currently known about such differences and preferences, except that they exist.

While many different kinds of living arrangements are possible, most elderly persons are limited in their choices and those with the least financial and family resources have the fewest options. Even public housing for the elderly discriminates against the functionally impaired (Carp 1976; Lawton 1969) and congregate housing and other alternatives are not often an option. An institution becomes the chief and perhaps the only alternative for most of the disabled low-income elderly without family support.

Policy Implications

The most important finding from the survey data, in our view, is the dominant influence of marital status and living arrangements on the risk of institutionalization. This confirms the findings of other research about the importance of nonhealth factors for long-term-care policy. The surprising element in the finding is a quantitative one. Health status is of relatively low significance compared with marital status and living arrangements as a factor in determining risk of institutionalization. Large numbers of persons living in the community are as healthy, measured by disability, as those who are in institutions. Those living alone have up to five times as great a chance of being institutionalized as married persons whose health generally is not as good.

A second significant finding, closely related to the first, flows from the unpublished data on various age groups within the over 65 population. The disability data show that classifying persons by age, using terms such as "frail elderly" and "old old," can be misleading. While the percentage of disabled increases with age, the increase is not abrupt, and it is accompanied by a decrease in total numbers. As a result, nearly three-fifths of the disabled elderly population at risk is under 75. And the percentage of those 75 and over who are at risk is not as high as might have been expected. Well over half of that group is healthy and needs, not more medical care, but continued income and other social support to live adequately.

A third finding concerns the dominance of chronic versus acute illness among all elderly and the particular kinds of chronic conditions from which they suffer. All of the leading conditions afflicting the elderly have the classic characteristics of chronic illness. Almost by definition these conditions are not curable given the present state of medical knowledge. They require continuing management to reduce acute flare-ups that lead to hospitalization and to maximize the period of remission characteristic of such conditions. Because of the psychological and social aspects of chronic illness, ranging from depression to dependency, proper management requires integrating medical treatment with other forms of support and care. Any policy that makes the proper management of the condition difficult, or emphasizes one aspect of care at the expense of others on which its success depends, is heading in the wrong direction.

Finally, the analysis reveals that income and race, as expected, are important social factors in determining who is at risk, and that region and residence are not as important. Judging from the survey data, no surprising social factors have been overlooked in other research. If there is a justification for the current long-term-care pattern in which nonwhites, Southerners, and rural residents are receiving fewer long-term-care services than others, it is not in the nature of the population at risk.

From these findings some conclusions can be drawn on specific policy questions concerning long-term care of the elderly.

Relative Priority of Social versus Medical Interventions

The balance in federal spending on the over 65 population is steadily tilting toward medical spending and away from spending for other social purposes. For example, in 1970, cash assistance (Old Age and Survivors

Insurance) through Social Security provided over $4 for every dollar spent for the elderly on medical services through Medicare. By 1978 that ratio had shrunk to less than $3 of cash assistance for every Medicare dollar for the elderly.

The importance of living arrangements and other social factors in the population at risk of institutionalization suggests that this shift in policy is unfortunate. Considering those persons most at risk, the disabled living alone, the chances that added medical spending will reduce the risk of institutionalization seem slight. Even if expanded medical care stabilizes a chronic condition through good management, the everyday problems of living with that condition still remain. In contrast, added dollars for housing, nutrition, and other services may assist the elderly in improving their lives and avoiding institutionalization.

Without some change in policy, we can expect the current shift in spending toward medical care to continue. Medical care prices, particularly in hospitals, are rising more rapidly than prices generally. Since cash assistance under Social Security and other forms of assistance to the elderly are not increasing as fast, the medical piece of the elderly "pie" is increasing with time. The ability of government to adjust other spending to compensate for this shift will decrease with time because the number of elderly is growing in relation to total population. For example, while the elderly already account for a large chunk of total national spending for hospital care (27.7 percent), their share will continue to increase to over 30 percent during the next 20 years and to over 40 percent by the year 2025 as the percentage of elderly in the population grows to a projected 17.3 percent. These estimates do not reflect the increase in the average age of the over-65 population, which will tend to accelerate growth in hospital expenditures even further.

In short, controlling the rate of increase in medical spending for the elderly seems essential to any improvement in policy addressed to their long-term care.

Policies Focused on a Particular Age Group

The finding that age is a somewhat misleading guide to health status has at least two major implications. One is that age 65 has no particular significance for long-term-care policy. The percentage of population at risk between 65 and 74 is not much greater than that of those between 55 and 64, considering the similar health status and marital status of the two groups. In our view both groups should have similar long-term-care benefits. Another implication is that persons over 75, and even over 85, do not require special consideration so much because they are frail and elderly but because they are the ones most apt to be alone. Policies designed to bring them together with others in supportive social situations are likely to be more effective than policies designed to give them special care, medical or otherwise.

Priorities within Medical Policy

The dominant influence of chronic conditions on the health status of the over 65 population, and the relatively high concentration of those conditions in a definable group of people, suggest some new directions for medical policy. Currently federal policy toward medical care of the elderly is focused on giving them, through health insurance of a traditional sort (Medicare), the financial ability to pay for care. At least three aspects of that approach make it relatively inappropriate to a population with a high concentration of chronic illness.

First, the coverage emphasizes episodic acute hospital care when the illnesses affecting the elderly require continuous management, ideally outside of hospitals. Second, insurance plans are financial devices, not programs for reaching out to identify the chronically ill and guiding them toward ongoing appropriate care for their particular condition. Since the elderly chronically ill are perhaps less able than any other group to seek out on their own the medical care most appropriate to them, many are bound to end up with inadequate care or unnecessary care. Third, the government is buying into a medical care system whose financial incentives and organization generally are not consistent with the proper management of chronic illness. The traditional fee-for-service, cost reimbursement method of payment, which Medicare uses, provides an incentive to deliver more care and more costly care. Rather than rewarding the proper management of chronic illness and the prevention of acute flare-ups requiring hospitalization, it can actually reward mismanagement by paying for the resulting more costly care. Thus, it provides no economic incentive to existing medical organizations to find ways to deliver continuing low-cost care of chronic conditions. It offers no impetus to medical providers to organize themselves to seek out the chronically ill elderly and to serve them appropriately and efficiently.

Conclusion

While there can be no one "right" answer in addressing the health and social factors influencing long-term care, one conclusion seems inescapable. The data do not justify the present mix of policies. Health factors are important but not important enough in our view to justify the present emphasis on medical care. The way we organize and pay for medical care does not fit the health problems of the elderly and should be modified.

The search for a new mix of policies might start with a different view of the needs from the one which equates age with illness. The population at risk for long-term care is not a homogeneous group of elderly all needing the same services and support. It is rather a collection of individuals of different ages with different medical problems, family situations, living conditions, and incomes. They ought to be served by policies and programs flexible enough to adjust to their special needs.

Appendix: Sources and Limitations of the Data

Information used in this paper is based primarily on data collected in the 1973, 1974, 1976, and 1977 Health Interview Surveys and the 1973–74 National Nursing Home Survey. Data from the Health Interview Survey (HIS) is collected in a continuing nationwide survey conducted by household interview. Each week a probability sample of households is interviewed by trained personnel of the U.S. Bureau of the Census to obtain information about the health and other characteristics of the civilian non-institutionalized population of the United States. Each year the sample is composed of approximately 40,000 households containing between 110,000 and 140,000 persons.

Data from the National Nursing Home Survey (NNHS) focused on a national sample of nursing homes that provided some level of nursing care during the survey period from August 1973 to April 1974. The NNHS sample include approximately 1,900 nursing homes. In each home data were collected for a sample of approximately 10 residents through personal interviews with members of the nursing staff familiar with the medical records and/or care provided to the residents.

As in all analyses of survey data, the estimates, inferences, and conclusions drawn in this paper are influenced by the limitations of the survey design. The estimates presented are influenced by the kinds of questions asked, and perhaps equally by the kinds of questions not asked. Similarly, how the survey terms are defined will affect the results. For example, if disability was defined differently, our estimates of the number of disabled elderly and our policy conclusions might be quite different. The interpretation of survey data in terms of the inferences and conclusions drawn is also affected by the authors' previous experiences, values, and biases. We have presented our view of the policy implications of the survey data, but suggest that each reader draw his or her own conclusions.

Since the statistics presented in this report are based on samples, they will differ somewhat from the figures that would have resulted had a complete census been taken of the target populations using the same schedules, instructions, and interviewing personnel and procedures. As in any survey or census, the results also are subject to reporting and processing errors, and errors due to nonresponse. Those errors are kept to a minimum by methods built into survey procedures. The nonresponse rates in general are quite low: about 4 percent for the HIS and about 2 percent for the resident questionnaire used on the NNHS. In addition, HIS estimates are adjusted within each of 60 age-sex-race cells to independent population estimates prepared by the Bureau of the Census for the survey period. The effect of this adjustment is to make the sample more closely representative of the population, thereby reducing error. However, with the exception of population estimates adjusted according to the process above, HIS estimates are based on the HIS household sample and will differ from figures (derived from different sources) published in reports of the Bureau of the Census.

Although sampling errors for most estimates presented in this paper are relatively small, in cases where the estimate (or the numerator or denominator of the estimate) is small, the sample error will be high. The National Center for Health Statistics standard of minimum reliability and precision for HIS estimates is that the standard error of the estimate not exceed 30 percent of the estimate itself; for the NNHS the standard is set at 25 percent. In cases where the standard errors exceed these estimates an asterisk is placed above the relevent estimate. In such cases the estimates should be interpreted with due caution.

One other methodological issue, that of the confounding effects of age, period, and cohort, should be raised. In empirical studies on aging, the apparent effects of aging (e.g., reduced health status) are almost always confounded with the effects of other variables associated with aging. That is, age differences are, in part, due to the different environmental histories of each age group or cohort and, in part, a function of the time that the measurement was taken. More specifically, the age-related variations in disability and other variables discussed in the text are the combined product of the effect of aging itself, or age effects; the effect of influences associated with the date of birth of population groups, or cohort effects; and the effect of the time period in which the observations are taken, or period effects. Unfortunately, there is no simple or straightforward statistical method for distinguishing among these effects.

In our view, the relevance of this issue for policy lies primarily in the future. That is, policies which are based on evidence regarding the current elderly cohort may not be appropriate for future elderly cohorts. The elderly of the future will have experienced different environmental histories and may have different needs.[4]

Table 2.16   **Institutionalization Rates for Elderly, U.S., 1973–74**

	Nursing Home Population[a]	Noninstitutionalized Population[b]	Estimated Institutionaliza-tion Rate/1000
65–74			
Married	30,100	8,087,300	4
Widowed	75,100	3,538,700	21
Alone	29,800	2,262,000	13
Relatives	41,000	1,169,400	34
Nonrelatives	4,300*	107,200	39
Never married/			
Div/Sep	57,900	1,345,600	41
Alone	20,700	762,300	26
Relatives	33,200	480,800	65
Nonrelatives	4,000*	102,400	38
75–84			
Married	54,800	2,648,800	20
Widowed	263,400	3,060,600	79
Alone	109,700	1,852,100	56
Relatives	145,200	1,105,800	116
Nonrelatives	8,400	102,600	76
Never married/			
Div/Sep	66,700	586,500	102
Alone	35,300	316,000	100
Relatives	27,800	222,900	111
Nonrelatives	3,600*	47,600	70
85+			
Married	32,200	252,400	113
Widowed	328,600	867,300	275
Alone	131,400	373,000	261
Relatives	188,400	454,600	293
Nonrelatives	8,800	39,700	181
Never married/			
Div/Sep	52,800	110,500	323
Alone	30,300	54,000	359
Relatives	19,100	43,400	306
Nonrelatives	3,500*	13,100*	211

[a]Estimates based on data from the 1973–74 National Nursing Home Survey
[b]Data from the 1973–74 Health Interview Survey
*Figure does not meet NCHS standards of reliability or precision.

Table 2.17	Institutionalization Rates for Male Elderly, U.S., 1973–74		
	Nursing Home Population[a]	Noninstitutionalized Population[b]	Estimated Institutionaliza-tion Rate/1000
65–74			
Married	15,600	4,540,800	3
Widowed	17,600	538,300	32
Alone	7,100	323,800	21
Relatives	8,700	190,400	44
Nonrelatives	1,800*	24,100*	69
Never married/			
Div/Sep	31,800	545,300	55
Alone	12,900	309,800	40
Relatives	17,800	183,700	88
Nonrelatives	1,100*	51,800	21
75–84			
Married	28,500	1,676,800	17
Widowed	46,900	552,600	78
Alone	20,600	310,500	62
Relatives	24,800	216,900	103
Nonrelatives	1,400*	25,200*	53
Never married/			
Div/Sep	26,900	208,800	114
Alone	14,800	109,600	119
Relatives	11,200	79,100	124
Nonrelatives	900*	20,100*	43
85+			
Married	18,900	187,500	92
Widowed	64,300	199,800	243
Alone	25,800	89,200	224
Relatives	37,400	105,300	262
Nonrelatives	1,200*	5,300*	185
Never married/			
Div/Sep	15,000	31,800	321
Alone	7,300*	15,500*	320
Relatives	5,900*	11,400*	341
Nonrelatives	1,700*	4,900*	258

[a]Estimates based on data from the 1973–74 National Nursing Home Survey
[b]Data from the 1973–74 Health Interview Survey
*Figure does not meet NCHS standards of reliability or precision.

Table 2.18	Institutionalization Rates for Female Elderly, U.S., 1973–74		
	Nursing Home Population[a]	**Noninstitutionalized Population**[b]	**Estimated Institutionaliza-tion Rate/1000**
65–74			
Married	14,500	3,546,500	4
Widowed	57,500	3,000,400	19
Alone	22,700	1,938,200	12
Relatives	32,200	979,100	32
Nonrelatives	2,600*	83,100	30
Never married/ Div/Sep	25,900	800,300	31
Alone	8,200	452,500	18
Relatives	15,200	297,100	49
Nonrelatives	2,500*	50,600	47
75–84			
Married	26,300	972,000	26
Widowed	216,500	2,507,900	79
Alone	89,200	1,541,600	55
Relatives	120,300	888,900	119
Nonrelatives	7,000	77,400	83
Never married/ Div/Sep	39,800	377,700	95
Alone	20,700	206,500	91
Relatives	16,500	143,800	103
Nonrelatives	2,600*	27,500	86
85+			
Married	13,300	64,800	170
Widowed	264,400	667,500	284
Alone	105,700	283,800	271
Relatives	151,200	349,300	302
Nonrelatives	7,600	34,400	181
Never married/ Div/Sep	37,500	78,700	323
Alone	22,400	38,500	368
Relatives	13,200	32,000	292
Nonrelatives	1,900*	8,200*	188

[a]Estimates based on the 1973–74 National Nursing Home Survey
[b]Data from the 1973–74 Health Interview Survey
*Figure does not meet NCHS standards for reliability or precision.

Notes

1. Responsibility for interpretation of the data is solely that of the authors. The analyses and conclusions do not necessarily reflect the views of the National Center for Health Statistics or the Administration on Aging.

2. For a description of the source and limitations of the data see the appendix.

3. Compared with other more sophisticated indexes of functional ability, the limitation of activity classification is relatively crude. Rather than assessing whether a chronic condition results in a limitation in a person's ability to perform school, work, housework, or social activities, these more sophisticated measures address a range of specific activities essential to daily living. For example, the Index of Activities of Daily Living (Katz, et al., 1963) measures ability to perform self-maintenance activities such as bathing, feeding, etc., while the Instrumental Activities of Daily Living Scale (Lawton and Brody 1969) extends beyond physical self-maintenance to such items as preparing meals, using a telephone, washing clothes, etc. Even more complex instruments such as the OARS Multidimensional Functional Assessment (Pfeiffer 1975) measure well-being in terms of social resources, economic resources, mental health, and physical health in addition to measuring activities of daily living. Unlike the limitation of activity classification used in HIS, these indexes offer the added advantage of measuring function independently of social roles, i.e., work other than labor force participation. Unfortunately, none of these more sophisticated measures has been used to date on a national scale.

4. For further discussion of these issues we refer the reader to N. Glenn, *Cohort Analysis* (Beverly Hills: Sage Publications, 1977), and G. Maddox and J. Wiley, "Scope, Concepts, and Methods in the Study of Aging," in *Handbook of Aging and Social Sciences,* ed. R. Binstock and E. Shanas (New York: Van Nostrand Reinhold, 1976).

Bibliography

Berg, Robert L., et al. "Assessing the Health Care Needs of the Aged." *Health Services Research* (Spring 1970), pp. 36–59.

Berkman, L., and Syme, S. "Social Networks, Host Resistance, and Mortality: A Nine-Year Follow-up Study of Alameda County Residents." *American Journal of Epidemiology* 109, no. 2 (1979).

Breslau, N., and Haug, M. "The Elderly Aid the Elderly: The Senior Friends Program." *Social Security Bulletin* 35 (1972), pp. 9–15.

Brockington, F., and Lempert, S. M. *The Social Needs of the Over-80s.* Manchester, Eng.: Manchester University Press, 1966.

Carp, F. "Housing and Living Environments of Older People," in *Handbook of Aging and the Social Sciences,* ed. R. Binstock and E. Shanas. New York: Van Nostrand Reinhold, 1976.

Davis, J., and Gibbon, M. "An Areawide Examination of Nursing Home Use, Misuse, and Nonuse." *American Journal of Public Health* 61, no. 6 (1971).

Dunlop, B. "Long-Term Care: Need Versus Utilization." Urban Institute Working Paper 0975-05, May 1974 (revised 1975).

Eggert, G. M., et al. "Caring for the Patient with Long-Term Disability." *Geriatrics,* October, 1977, pp. 102–14.

Haber, L. D. "Identifying the Disabled: Concepts and Methods in the Measurement of Disability." *Social Security Bulletin* 30, no. 12 (December, 1967): 17–35.

Haberstein, R. W., and Biddle, E. W. "Decision to Relocate the Residence of Aged Persons." Center for Research in Social Behavior, University of Missouri, Columbus, January 1974.

Katz, E., et al. "Studies of Illness in the Aged. The Index of ADL: A Standardized Measure of Biological and Psychosocial Function." *Journal of the American Medical Association* 185, no. 12, (1963).

Kelly, L. "Consistency of the Adult Personality." *American Psychologist* 10 (1955).

Kovar, M. G. "Health of the Elderly and the Use of Health Services." *Public Health Reports* 92, no. 1 (January–February 1977): 9–19.

Lawrence, Philip S. "Patterns of Health and Illness in Older People." *Bulletin of the NY Academy of Medicine* 49, no. 12 (December 1973): 1100–1109.

Lawton, M. P. "Supportive Services in the Context of the Housing Environment." *Gerontologist* 9 (1969).

Lawton, M. P. "The Functional Assessment of Elderly People." *Journal of the American Geriatric Society* 19 (June 1971): 465–81.

Lawton, M. P., and Brody, E. M. "Assessment of Older People: Self-Maintaining and Instrumental Activities of Daily Living." *Gerontologist* 9, no. 5 (Autumn 1969), pt. 1.

Litman, T. J. "Health Care and the Family: A Three-Generational Analysis." *Medical Care* 9 (1971).

Lowenthal, M. F., and Robinson, B. "Social Networks and Isolation." In *Handbook of Aging and the Social Sciences*, ed. R. Binstock and E. Shanas. New York: Van Nostrand Reinhold, 1976.

Maddox, G. L. "Self-Assessment of Health Status: A Longitudinal Study of Selected Elderly Subjects." *Journal of Chronic Disease* 17 (May 1964): 449–60.

Maddox, G. L., and Douglass, E. B. "Self-Assessment of Health: A Longitudinal Study of Elderly Subjects." *Journal of Health and Social Behavior* 14 (1973): 87–93.

McCoy, John L., and Brown, David L. "Health Status among Low-Income Elderly Persons: Rural-Urban Differences." *Social Security Bulletin* 41, no. 6 (June 1978): 14–26.

National Center for Health Statistics (NCHS). *Limitations of Activity Due to Chronic Conditions*. DHEW Publ. No. (HRA) 77-1537, Series 10, No. 111. Rockville, Maryland: U.S. Department of Health, Education, and Welfare, 1977*a*.

National Center for Health Statistics (NCHS). *Utilization of Nursing Homes: United States National Nursing Home Survey, August 1973–April 1974*. DHEW Publ. No. (HRA) 77-1779, Series 13, No. 28. Hyattsville, Maryland: U.S. Department of Health, Education, and Welfare, 1977*b*.

National Center for Health Statistics (NCHS). *Current Estimates from the Health Interview Survey*. DHEW Publ. No. (PHS) 78-1554, Series 10, No. 126. Rockville, Maryland: U.S. Department of Health, Education, and Welfare, 1978.

Palmore, E. "Total Chance of Institutionalization among the Aged." *Gerontologist* 16, no. 6 (1976).

Pfeiffer, Eric, ed. *Multidimensional Functional Assessment: The OARS Methodology, A Manual*. Center for the Study of Aging and Human Development, Duke University, Durham, North Carolina, 1975.

Scanlon, W. "Nursing Home Utilization Patterns: Implications for Policy." Urban Institute Working Paper: 5904-10, April, 1978.

Shanas, E. *The Health of Older People: A Social Survey*. Cambridge, Mass.: Harvard University Press, 1962.

Shanas, E., et al. *Old People in Three Industrial Societies*. New York: Aldine, 1968.

Shanas, E. "Measuring the Home Health Needs of the Elderly in Five Countries." *Journal of Gerontology* 26 (1971):37–40.

Shanas, E. "The Family as a Social Support System in Old Age." *Gerontologist* 19, no. 2 (1979).

Shanas, E., and Maddox, G. L. "Aging, Health, and the Organization of Health Resources," in *Handbook of Aging and the Social Sciences,* ed. R. Binstock and E. Shanas. New York: Van Nostrand Reinhold, 1976.

Sussman, M. "The Family Life of Old People," in *Handbook of Aging and the Social Sciences,* ed. R. Binstock and E. Shanas. New York: Van Nostrand Reinhold, 1976.

World Health Organization, Regional Office for Europe. *The Public Health Aspects of the Aging of the Population,* 1959.

3. The Extent and Nature of Public Responsibility for Long-Term Care

Robert L. Kane and Rosalie A. Kane

Introduction

Those who survive into old age are at high risk of developing multiple physical and social problems, which threaten their very ability to exist independently. Long-term care (LTC) refers to the composite of health and social services needed to sustain such persons. In this paper we examine the way our society has approached its responsibility toward this care to ask some fundamental questions about the nature of this responsibility: Should some assistance with basic care be guaranteed to each citizen in his old age? On whose terms should LTC be offered?

At the outset, let us consider the typical problems of the candidate for LTC. These are best depicted not as complicated medical diagnoses, but as common, unglamorous problems that render elderly persons dependent on others. In functional terms, the major problems are immobility, falls, incontinence, and mental disturbances (often labeled dementia). These difficulties, which may occur singly or in combination, are the ones most likely to cause dependency on other human beings for satisfaction of basic needs for food, shelter, cleanliness, and safety.

At present much of the long-term care offered in the United States is being provided in institutional, hospitallike settings, primarily in nursing homes. Conceivably the necessary attention could also be provided to people in their own homes. For each nursing home resident who is incontinent, immobile, or disoriented, about two with the same degree of disability are being managed in the community through the use of personal and/or family resources (U.S. Comptroller General 1979). As public re-

This paper was prepared as part of a project directed by the University of Chicago School of Social Service Administration and sponsored by the Administration on Aging.

An early draft of this paper was reviewed by a number of individuals. We would like to thank them for their very useful suggestions and criticisms, but the authors take public responsibility for the final product. Our thanks go to the following: Ruth Covell, John Flanagan, Christopher Foote, Charles Levy, Joseph Newhouse, and Florence Patton.

sponsibility for LTC is considered, some decisions are required about basic priorities. For example, is the society responsible for identifying and offering care to those managing on their own, or is it sufficient to supply care on request? To what extent can conditions be placed on the benefits received, particularly extreme conditions that might require relocating in an institution? To what extent is there a public obligation to treat vigorously, manage, and study problems such as falls, incontinence, and dementia so that symptoms can be reversed when possible or their effects minimized? Should each stroke patient receive intensive rehabilitation?

The shape of public policy toward long-term care, especially its financing, may well require a change in public attitudes toward the aged and the aging process. We have tended to focus our discussions and our programs on that segment of the aged population that is dependent. It is equally necessary to underscore that there is a larger segment who are not dependent or who are disabled but manage without major reliance on public programs. At a minimum we note that those surviving into old age are healthier than earlier generations. Controlling for age, the elderly of today are fitter than their forebears.

Furthermore, when we provide LTC, whether vigorously investigative and therapeutic or passively custodial and protective, to what extent should family resources be tapped before public help is offered? Is the object of policy to relieve burdens of families or is it to provide residual care when family assistance is impractical? On the other side of the coin, to what extent should public policy protect the elderly from either exploitation or well-meaning overprotection by family and friends? Such questions must be addressed as part of efforts to define public responsibility for long-term care.

A Question of Values

Current conceptions of public responsibility for long-term care are reflected in present programs and policies and the statements of those who would restructure these public programs. Any scrutiny of public responsibility takes on moral overtones, raising debate about what ought to be the nature and extent of public provisions compared with the responsibility of individuals, families, and private philanthropy. Ultimately such judgments—not only about the relative importance of particular problems and the relative worth of vulnerable populations that compete for a share of finite resources, but also about the very nature of the social order and the proper divisions between public and private responsibility—are based on values.

Because our subject involves elements of a moral discourse, we begin by clarifying what we mean by values. Values are simply preferences held by individuals or groups. In considering long-term care, for example, various public servants, professional groups, or human service organizations have views about desirable outcomes of programs and preferred ways of achieving such outcomes. In other words, both means and ends are matters of value judgment. Because values are beliefs, it is inappropriate to study whether values espoused by any group are correct. Still, a major policy issue revolves around the question of whose values are used to shape policy.

For the most part, studies related to values fall into three general categories: (1) surveys conducted to describe or rank preferred values of the public or of various subgroups; (2) studies to assess the effectiveness of programs developed to achieve valued objectives; and (3) studies evaluating the value implications of programs, i.e., predicting or demonstrating the outcomes of different policies so that choices can be made on the basis of the most valued outcomes. In all these categories, value-related research in LTC remains largely undone.

Values should not be confused with ethics, which are standards of behavior that are derived from values. As Levy (1976) indicates, ethics are codified values. Serious ethical dilemmas involving nursing home care, quality of life of the aged, and treatment of the terminally ill have been cited by those calling for a fresh approach to health ethics. Yet ethical behavior is difficult to define when underlying values are unclear. Only when public responsibility for long-term care is better articulated (as a result of clarification of basic social values), can ethical practice be better specified for those institutions and workers concerned with LTC delivery.

Perspectives on Public Responsibility

Public policy regarding LTC can be examined from several perspectives, namely, (1) articulation of goals, which constitutes an official statement of desired events, (2) allocation of resources to bring about those desired events, and (3) analysis of areas of omission. As many commentators have indicated, policy development, particularly in long-term care, is a fragmented responsibility and has produced confusing, and at times inconsistent, entitlements. Implementation of policy is similarly decentralized and diffuse. Binstock and Levin (1976) distinguish policy adoption from policy implementation; both must be considered in a description of the extent and nature of public programming. The multiplicity of public actors in the long-term-care field complicates any discussion of public responsibility.

Perhaps the most serious complexity is introduced into the subject by the vagueness of the goals espoused. Long-term-care policy, like most social policy, is a product of compromise. When goals are articulated at a very general level, however, divisions of opinion are glossed over. For example, substantial agreement could be reached that long-term care should promote independent functioning of persons with chronic impairments and provide the conditions under which they can enjoy a good quality of life. Once discussion leaves this elevated plane, serious disagreements may emerge among people nominally committed to achieving the same goals.

Disagreements about goals may take several forms. First, disagreements often develop over operational definitions. There is little agreement on the meaning of terms such as, for example, independence. Second, disagreements may concern the relative priority to be assigned to alternative goals. Finally, differences on other basic social values could lead to profoundly different expectations about programming to achieve long-term goals. For instance, a person committed to governmental regulation might take a very different approach to guaranteeing a high quality of life for the nursing home patient than a person committed to free market devices. Other important social values pertinent to one's view of public responsibility for LTC would include views on the appropriate roles of nuclear and extended families, states' rights as opposed to federal government, institutional versus community living, and even basic convictions about the extent to which government should be involved in the life of the private citizen.

Because human service programs represent uneasy compromises among diverse interests and values, their official goals are characteristically vague (Hasenfeld and English 1974). Serious exploration of public responsibility for LTC must go beyond official rhetoric to a discussion of specific desired outcomes and their implications. In this paper we examine public responsibility as a concept, discussing various rationales that might underlie different public policies, the goals of such policies, and the multiple public roles that have been taken and could be taken in relation to LTC. When possible, we anchor our discussion with specific examples. In the last section we return to the value issues where we began. We maintain that public discussion about public responsibility for long-term care is enormously important. Without clear statements about the purpose of public LTC provisions, an evaluator cannot determine whether the public's will is being done. Also, unless the exercise of public responsibility is deliberate and planful, we are at risk of supporting a policy with a low likelihood of achieving the outcomes that are publicly valued.

Definition
Public

The concept of "public" may be construed from several, potentially overlapping, perspectives. Perhaps the source of greatest confusion is that the term may refer both to things popular, i.e., in the domain of the

general populace, and also somewhat more narrowly to things governmental, i.e., to the theoretical instrument of that populace. When we
address issues of responsibility, we use the term "public" in the latter
context to distinguish those activities and responsibilities which are, and
may be governmental from those that are private.

Long-Term Care

Earlier in this volume our colleagues introduced a definition of long-term
care. Like most definitions of LTC, it includes physical and emotional
care (apart from the care of a normally developing child) provided over a
sustained period of time for those incapable of sustaining themselves
without that care. In the context of a discussion of public responsibility
for LTC, it is particularly important that the term be defined independently of present solutions. Operationally, LTC in the United States
is often viewed as care given to those served in nursing homes or, conversely, services designed to keep them outside such institutions. Despite
the broadness of accepted definitions, too often the nursing home becomes the automatic focus of discussions about LTC policy.

A discussion of public responsibility demands exploring the implications of the definition. The boundaries that interested parties place
around a definition provide an early indication of how responsibility is
construed. What, for example, is meant by a sustained period of time?
LTC is differentiated from acute care because the latter involves only a
predictably brief period of dependency, but what is the cutoff point? We
consider LTC to be care required for a period of a month or more, but a
different construction of the problem would lead to a different formulation
of the solution. In fact, LTC needs may include a continuous need for a
minimal level of service interspersed with cyclical or periodic needs for
intensive care such as that usually associated with the acute sector.

Our definition leaves a number of points imprecise. The provider of
LTC, for example, is deliberately not specified, allowing for both formal
and informal provision of services. LTC can be provided by family and
friends of the recipient as well as by institutions and agencies. Also open
is the issue of financing; LTC may be funded by the recipient or his
family, by private philanthropy or public dollars. The time of family
members and unrelated volunteers is also part of the LTC cost.

A chronic illness (such as arthritis) or a disability (such as deafness)
may not necessitate long-term care. Only when the problem grows beyond the capacity of the individual to manage without physical assistance
or personal care of others is LTC relevant. Whether an individual with a
given physical problem will require LTC may depend on individual moti-
vational and psychological factors as well as on the physical condition
itself.

LTC needs differ in both intensity and duration. Some problems require a period of care that is short and predictable—e.g., a fractured hip rendering an individual dependent for two or three months. Other problems may necessitate nursing care or special protection for the remainder of a lifetime. Sometimes care needs are minimal—e.g., assitance with transportation or with heavy tasks. Sometimes they are extensive—e.g., complete assistance with dressing, bathing, and feeding. A great many degrees of need fall between these two extremes.

Isaacs and Neville (1975, 1976) developed a practical classification system to determine the nature of LTC need based on the length of the interval between episodes of necessary help. Need was considered minimal if help was required with heavy tasks performed infrequently (such as shopping or heavy cleaning); long-interval need requirements involved a need for help every 24 hours or longer; short-interval need described requirements for assistance every few hours during the day; and critical interval need was used to describe the need for the constant presence of another individual because requirements for help are frequent and unpredictable. As a subsequent step in describing unmet need, Isaacs also classified the patterns of solitude of elderly individuals in a fourfold system; minimal solitude for those rarely alone (usually living with a spouse or child); diurnal for those alone much of the day but not at night; nocturnal for those alone at night but with access to others at regular intervals during the day; and maximal for those almost entirely alone. Obviously the individual with short interval needs and maximum solitude is lacking in needed basic care.

The importance of such classification systems is their ability to identify patterns in the mix between need and availability of care, which, in turn, suggest differing packages of services to keep the individual maximally independent. For example, day care is relevant for those with diurnal solitude and high needs, while night sitting might be more important for those with nocturnal solitude. Other promising formulations have been developed by the Community Council of Greater New York (1978) and by Grauer and Birnbom in Montreal (1975).

With such classification systems, public responsibility could be differentially defined depending on the duration and intensity of need. For example, those with limited need for infrequent care might be eligible for care at home whereas those requiring care exceeding a certain threshold could be required to receive it only in an institutional setting. In another example, the individual might be held responsible for payment for minimal service, whereas intensive services would be covered as part of a benefit package. At present, nursing home care coverage is an entitlement for elderly citizens regardless of income only when it is required for a brief, posthospital recuperative period. Otherwise payment for nursing home care is not a public responsibility unless the recipient has exhausted his resources and is officially "poor." Of course another, and arguably preferable, way of defining public responsibility would be to emphasize home care as the goal of choice in all instances, regardless of the efficiency of such care compared with institutional settings.

Need for LTC implies dependency, which may also be of several kinds. Direct dependency on the personal services of others occurs in all income groups. Economic dependency by itself (which, not surprisingly, overtakes the poor first) can give rise to other dependencies. For example, some individuals could function without direct personal services if they could purchase the equipment and environmental supports needed. LTC recipients also vary in the amount and kinds of skills on which they depend; some may be dependent on advanced technological care for survival, whereas others may need less-specialized services such as help with laundry or homemaking.

We referred to LTC as sustained physical or emotional care. Although debates sometimes occur about whether LTC is a social or a medical service, the distinction is really artificial. Physical care is usually a necessary but insufficient component of the service. In fact, physical needs are so responsive to psychological and social factors that it is almost impossible to separate the two. Dependency can be created or exacerbated because of psychological factors such as fear, depression, or anxiety, and these, in turn, are influenced by social factors such as family relationships or the safety of the neighborhood.

Candidates for LTC

To summarize our discussion of the long-term-care definition, we have emphasized that LTC is physical and social care provided over a sustained period of time for those incapable of functioning without such care. LTC can vary along a number of dimensions: duration, extent, source, and level of skilled input required.

A decision about the appropriate extent and nature of public programming for LTC depends on an analysis of the extent of need in the population. Unfortunately, predictions about LTC depends on an analysis of the extent of need in the population. Unfortunately, predictions about LTC needs, even in aggregate, are necessarily tentative and are likely to be relative to society's circumstances. For groups with a medical problem or condition, some predictions about the average length of expected long-term care can be made and some estimations of the types and intensity of care to improve the course of the patient could be hazarded, but their reliability is poor (Sager 1978). Such an exercise would yield an estimation of the total resources required for nursing and medical care. However, it is extremely difficult to make predictions about how much care an individual person with a given condition will require.

Furthermore, the public solution chosen will interact with the problem and perhaps change the prognosis of continued need. As already stated, for every person currently in a nursing home, two people in the community are equally disabled. If community-based care were widely available and attractively delivered, one might expect a more widespread utilization by the population in need. Moreover, there is some concern about creating an iatrogenic effect; the very provision of institutional care may cause a prolonged need for LTC. (This is especially true if policies encourage the burning of social bridges upon entry into an LTC facility.)

Our predictive skills are particularly poor in the area of prevention; we do not know to what extent provision of preventive health and social services (particularly companionship and recreation) prevents exacerbations and the need for more intensive levels of care in the future. Because the number of persons technically eligible for social care at such minimal levels would be astronomical, careful decisions would be needed based on knowledge about its benefit.

Any enumeration of the population at risk for LTC must take into account LTC that is provided (with or without TLC) by family members. In estimating the numbers of persons who would take advantage of a new entitlement (e.g., for housekeeping services apart from a medical problem), one must assume that some of those presently "making do" in the community would avail themselves of the new service. Pollak (1979) has cogently discussed the reasons why any policy directed at preventing institutionalization would have a much wider clientele than those persons currently admitted to nursing homes.

Long-term care has been appropriately defined in an open-ended and expansive way. Public policy, however, will need to be directed at clearly specified groups of people with provisions for eligibility requirements and gatekeeping functions. On precisely this point—i.e., how much the public should be expected to provide for what people—the value-laden debate must center.

Public and Private

In this paper, the term "public" is used synonymously with governmental. When we refer to public LTC policies, we are including the goals and actions of legislative, administrative, and judicial bodies at all governmental levels. Governmental action (or inaction) can affect the behavior of individual older persons and their families. Public programming also has great influence on the rise and decline of occupational groups. Undoubtedly, public LTC policy will powerfully affect a wide range of business enterprises and entrepreneurs with interests in providing long-term care.

The obvious opposite of public is private. In an age of worry over spiraling costs, encroaching government, and breakdown of the social order, public policies on LTC exert direct influence on three distinctive facets of the private sector: (1) personal; (2) philanthropic or nonprofit; and (3) proprietary or profit making. Each of these facets represents an aspect of LTC delivery, and public responsibility should be explicated in relation to the desired roles of these private systems. In a later section of this paper we discuss a variety of governmental roles in relation to LTC and for each one we allude to the implications for the private sphere.

Each of our three "private worlds" is extremely important to LTC delivery. The private/personal is crucial because much LTC is currently provided through purchases by the individual and the literal caretaking of family members. The fear of opening a Pandora's box of expanded benefits and thereby disrupting the silent providers of nonreimbursed care (Pollak 1979) must be balanced against data that suggest that some public help is needed so that more families can continue providing care for longer periods of time rather than relinquishing the job to the government (Eggert, et al., 1975). Government action will cause family reaction. Many decisions are made on the basis of incentives for individuals and families. Such incentives may have profound implications for encouraging various kinds of intergenerational relationships.

Private philanthropic efforts are particularly important in LTC because of the pivotal volunteer services. LTC is manpower intensive. Public responsibility, broadly defined, may depend on the availability of volunteer assistance from neighbors, church and civic groups, and public interest organizations.

Finally, LTC users provide a ready market for private profit-making care providers. Self-employed workers, proprietary organizations, and chains of organizations will be encouraged or discouraged, expand, entrench, or diversify in response to public decisions about the amount and type of LTC benefits the government should provide. As we consider various public responses and initiatives in long-term care, each must be viewed in relation to its impact on private nonprofit and profit-making LTC provision. Again, policy should develop from a careful analysis of the advantages and disadvantages of stimulating nongovernmental services; conceivably, different decisions may be made in different program areas.

The development of a private sector which includes both paid and unpaid provision of LTC appears an essential part of any program for such care. It is both necessary and desirable that there be a system of care independent of the government. In this country, the majority of care is not rendered by public providers. Even in more socialized nations where public delivery is more modal, the presence of an alternative system is held desirable.

Similarly, the quality of service provided cannot depend solely on the extent to which behaviors are codified and those codes enforced. Health and social services are too complex to be readily regulated by an implicit list of prescribed and proscribed activities. The quality of care will be determined in fair measure by the professional standards and expectations of the providers. In some cases, the care will be good despite regulations rather than because of them.

Rationale for a Public LTC Policy
Constituencies

An LTC policy serves many masters. The most obvious beneficiary is the older population itself. A second constituency is the family of the older person, whose interests may not be identical to those of its elderly member. Third, the LTC industry itself benefits or suffers as a result of public decisions. Finally, the general public, personified by the taxpayer, also has a vital stake in the extent and nature of the government's responsibility for LTC. Out of these multiple, often overlapping interests, a coherent statement of public responsibility must be forged.

The Elderly.—The elderly population is not homogeneous. To assert what the elderly themselves would desire in an LTC policy requires a rather high level of generalization to embrace all the subgroups of the aged. In general, however, older persons expect an LTC program to provide required care in a way that preserves as much independence, autonomy, and choice as possible. Quite reasonably, they prefer to obtain such care without reducing their standard of living to the poverty level or depleting their estates. Institutional placement is widely dreaded as a fearsome event.

The particular expectations and preferences of any given generation of elderly persons are related to their age cohort as well as their age (Riley, et al., 1969). Thus, individuals in their 70s in the 1970s might believe that the attention of a personal physician is an indispensable attribute of good care and experience a sense of abandonment and deprivation if they do not perceive that they have access to such medical care, but subsequent cohorts of older persons may not share that value. Because the preferences of any group are a product of both their chronological age and their generational cohort status, research findings on value preferences of the elderly do not lend themselves readily to extrapolation to future groups of aged persons.

Some research is under way at present to determine what the older person regards as essential to a high quality of life (Flanagan 1978; Reid and Zeigler 1978). The nursing home itself seems to be an almost universal object of dread, and a fairly safe generalization is that older persons do not want to receive care in an institution. Other data suggest that elderly persons of all socioeconomic classes prefer to live independently of their children (Hill 1963).

Although age 65 has been reified by current public policy, it does not divide the population in any meaningful way. A 65-year-old may have more in common with a 55-year-old than with an 80-year-old. Verbal, politically aroused groups struggling against ageism may have few aspirations in common with older, more debilitated groups. Also, ethnic and economic distinctions create subgroups within the large group of elderly and give rise to differing needs and expectations. Finally, a substantial number of LTC candidates have been deemed impaired in judgment to the extent that they cannot manage their own affairs. It is difficult to determine the value preferences of such persons and even more difficult to decide what priority to give their choices.

The generation currently in its mid-40s to 50s is often the only economically productive generation in a four- or five-generation family (Beattie 1976). This stark statement emphasizes that the family is an interested beneficiary of any long-term-care policy. Generalizing about preferences of families is subject to the same caveats as generalizing about the preferences of the elderly. The family perspective may differ somewhat in emphasis from the perspective of the primary recipient. One could posit that the rationale for an LTC policy from a family perspective would be to provide for the adequate care of the elderly person while minimizing family expenditures, burdens, and guilt. As has been repeatedly demonstrated (Brody 1978; Shanas 1979), families have not abandoned the elderly and, in fact, are distressed when they are forced to relegate their care to others, particularly institutions. Unable to provide daily care themselves, sometimes because of lack of physical proximity and sometimes because all adult relatives are in the labor market, families sometimes become fearful for the safety of their relatives and advocate a more restrictive environment than the elderly person would prefer.

Families and family responsibility are sometimes discussed as though the only relevant family members are adult children. Spouses and siblings of the elderly person are equally important family members, involved in the provision and receipt of informal LTC. Such family members ask that an LTC policy not disrupt the family unit or force the whole family group into poverty to care for the needs of one of its members.

At the same time, the aged are, in a sense, in competition with those in younger cohorts who need social and medical services. Although a larger population of the aged than of younger groups needs such services, the absolute number of dependent younger persons is much larger. It is thus not clear whether the dependent elderly will find their purposes best served by aligning themselves with the aged as a block or with those also dependent but younger. The political potency of these alternative alignments is yet to be explored.

Not only are the needs and demands of other segments of society competing with those of the population in need of or at risk of LTC, but one might argue that an investment in the younger, more fit elements of society is an investment in the elderly of the future. Clinicians note that the elderly of today are generally fitter than those of the same age in generations past. In part, such trends have rendered anachronistic our traditional definitions of time-determined old age. The improved status of those entering old age today can be attributed to better social and environmental conditions and, possibly, to improved health care as well (McKeown 1976). Certainly one goal of our society would be that people enter old age in as fit condition as possible in order to delay the need for LTC. It is less clear whether the efforts to attain that end should be classified as programs.

The Industry.—Providers of care are important consumers of LTC policy and active advocates for policies favoring their interests. Although the rationale for a policy must be cast in terms of its primary beneficiaries, the industry itself has vested interests that may link us to expensive or undesirable solutions. Those belonging to what Estes (1979) has labeled "the Aging Enterprise" include both the proprietary and nonprofit providers of LTC services and the large host of professionals and nonprofessionals who are employed in the many nooks and crannies of the aging network.

The professionals and entrepreneurs who have invested (either literally or figuratively) in LTC provision are active and often vocal spokespersons for public policy that will serve the industry. As that industry expands, the force it exerts on policy also increases. The direct interests of long-term-care beneficiaries, in contrast, are less likely to be clearly articulated because of their heterogeneity as well as the vulnerability of the populations involved. Although a coherent LTC policy based on expressed public values has not yet been developed, public programs of the past several decades have subsidized the growth of a substantial private industry. Any efforts now to forge a comprehensive policy must take the existence and reactions of the industry into account.

The Taxpayer.—A recent Harris poll of the general public (Harris 1975) showed a high degree of acceptance of the concept that the government should take major responsibility for ensuring the well-being of retired citizens. The respondents overwhelmingly agreed with statements indicating that Social Security payments should rise with the cost of living and that the government should be involved in providing long-term care. Over 75 percent of the respondents endorsed the nonjudgmental view that the elderly are entitled to a dignified standard of care and living regardless of how much they earned during their working years. Of course, such public views are usually gathered in a context that does not require the respondent to consider the costs.

Such sentiments suggest widespread recognition that LTC is a public responsibility. The rationale for an LTC policy may be different for the average taxpayer than for the elderly potential recipient. The taxpayer may seek a policy that keeps the total tax burden as light as possible and that is, above all, fair. A fair or equitable policy implies equity of benefits among elderly beneficiaries and among the elderly constituency and other groups for whom a public responsibility exists. Equity among the elderly could be construed as simple equity (that is, an equal amount of benefits for each elderly person) or, more reasonably, equity based on need (that is, provision of care so that each will have an equal opportunity for independence or whatever other goal is established). If the latter construction of equity is used, as Callahan (1977) has discussed in another context, disproportionate amounts of benefits will be expended on individuals with the greatest needs.

Despite the public acceptance of programming for the elderly, some gerontologists fear a backlash of resentment about the proportion of resources already consumed by the elderly. Hudson (1978) notes that the share of public dollars expended on care of the elderly is growing at a more rapid rate than the proportion for any other group. In advancing a statement about public responsibility for LTC that will be acceptable to the taxpayer, the legitimate needs of other groups must be taken into account.

Goals

We have already indicated that there may be more consensus on a general level of goal statements than on specific identification of points to be achieved. Even at the more general conceptual level, however, goals for long-term-care programs are not clearly promulgated. Like many other areas of social policy, LTC policy is fraught with potentially inconsistent, and perhaps even overtly contradictory, goal statements. Policies on long-term care are particularly likely to be cast in terms of the World Health Organization's definition of health, which seeks to maximize social, physical, and mental well-being, apparently simultaneously. In the realm of long-term care, some goals express aspirations such as improved quality of life, physical health, or functional ability, at the same time that other goals deal with such outcomes as happiness, family involvement across generations, prolongation of life, and even high quality of death.

At times we must examine each goal more minutely or perhaps choose among competing goals. It is not always clear, for example, when it is appropriate to improve an individual's functional ability beyond that level that he, himself, would seek. If an individual exists in some state of equilibrium, to what extent is it appropriate to threaten to disrupt that state by active case finding? If, indeed, happiness is determined in part by an individual's expectations, do we serve that individual by raising those expectations? Or, to take another example, should one maximize physical safety for the infirm at the cost of a sterile, hospitallike environment without privacy or choice?

These are not simply idle questions to be raised at scholarly symposia. National statistics provide data that at least reflect this dilemma. Whereas almost 70 percent of the noninstitutionalized elderly report their health status as excellent or good, about 47 percent of these individuals are limited in activities by chronic conditions; only 14 percent are aware of no chronic conditions. The perception of illness may, therefore, depend upon whether one looks at it through the eyes of the professional or the client. From the professional standpoint, active detection and treatment of disease may lead to amelioration of symptoms, if not to prolonged survival. Active rehabilitation may increase mobility and decrease further deterioration. These undertakings, however, may be accomplished at the cost of pain, suffering, and disruption. Moreover, once an individual enters into the treatment system, it is often hard to abort the process. Despite professional enthusiasm, many of the treatments promoted may not be as efficacious as their advocates hope, nor do they achieve anticipated savings in overall costs (Weissert, Wan, and Livieratos 1979). The physical and emotional side effects must be considered as well as the general threat of promoting increased disability and dependency.

Multiple Public Roles

As we have suggested, public and private responsibilities exist in a state of regularly recalibrated equilibrium. Private initiative responds to public cues offered by funding sources and also to the need to provide uncovered services. Public responsibility for long-term care can, in part, be defined as filling in the voids not met by other systems, both formal and informal. The public agencies have a variety of strategies available to meet their multiple responsibilities. Beyond the provision of direct services, they can also stimulate the activities of others and monitor those activities once under way. We propose an alliterative typology of the various roles that might be played by different levels of government as a potential menu from which items may be selected for inclusion or exclusion or for pursuit at various levels of intensity. Such multiple roles might include: pensioning, purchasing, providing, policing, protecting, preventing, peopling, promoting, policymaking/priority setting and planning.

Pensioning

In most parts of the developed Western world it is accepted as a public responsibility that some form of economic security be provided for elderly individuals. The proportion of direct government pensions to private pensions varies among societies, but public responsibility consistently includes assuring that at least some minimum standard of living can be guaranteed. In the United States, we rely upon a mixed approach, which includes a government-operated pension fund (Social Security), encouragement of private pension support through tax incentives, and means-tested welfare payments through Supplemental Social Insurance (SSI).

The higher the level of income maintenance through pensioning, the greater is the individual's ability to purchase LTC services without the need for specific governmental programs to underwrite these costs. Some would argue that this is the most appropriate role for the government because it leaves the individual free to choose among a variety of uses for his funds. Others hasten to point out that the distribution of needs is not uniform and, therefore, any pension system would put an undue burden on those stricken with a severe need for sustained long-term care. In this context we note that, ironically, LTC, which may represent the greatest medical catastrophe in terms of financial drain on the victims, is virtually universally excluded from any discussions about a catastrophic health program.

Long-term care is truly a catastrophe. In an analysis of catastrophic health expenditures ($5,000 or more in 1974), individuals in nursing homes, psychiatric hospitals, and chronic and tuberculosis hospitals accounted for almost half of all catastrophic expenses (nursing homes accounted for 59 percent of these costs). Birnbaum (1978) observes, "This concentration of expense implies that catastrophic illness is as much a long-term care problem as an acute care problem, and is especially noteworthy in light of the general exclusion of those expenses from national health insurance proposals."

Because pensioning will not suffice to provide adequate security for the individual in times of need, other public roles must be considered. A definitive public policy must grapple with the extent to which a pension system should be independent of other LTC benefits provision. For example, if an individual enters a chronic hospital, should his pension support be reduced to reflect the fact that room and board are provided in the institution? Although it seems a logical policy to avoid duplication of benefits, the implications are that individuals may not be able to afford their rents or the upkeep of their homes once admitted to an institution. This gives institutional care an ominous finality, rendering impractical brief admissions for rehabilitation, relief of relatives, or short trial admissions to a residential facjlity. Similarly, if pensioning systems for husband and wife are linked, anomalies can occur; for example, if one spouse is to make use of institutional benefits under Medicaid, the other spouse may not only need to "spend down" to Medicaid level but also lose Social Security benefits (Pollak 1979).

Purchasing

It is as a purchaser of LTC services that government (particularly the federal government) currently plays a predominant role. Analysis of federal funding programs shows that the shape of these efforts creates strong incentives for institutional care (U.S. Comptroller General 1979). Substantial sums of money are involved in the purchase of institutional services from the private sector; in 1977, $7.2 billion in public funds was paid to nursing homes, and the majority of this expenditure was on behalf of elderly patients. This sum represents 57 percent of the total nursing home bill and 12 percent of the public funds spent in personal health care (Gibson and Fisher 1979). The rules for eligibility and the scope of purchased services vary from program to program; governmental units purchase services from each other and from the nonprofit voluntary sector as well as from proprietary organizations. Purchase of care from family members and neighbors occurs less frequently. There seems to be a view that it is somehow wrong to reimburse persons for fulfilling family duties, despite the fact that family members lose income opportunities when delivering extensive LTC.

The levels of reimbursement and the eligibility for payment will directly affect the way care is given. The incentives for nursing home care over home care, or even other forms of sheltered care, have been well documented (U.S. Comptroller General 1979). Where a primary goal is cost containment, the restricted payments to nursing homes may all but preclude any efforts to upgrade care.

The Medicare program is designed as an entitlement program for individuals 65 years of age and older (as well as for other chronically disabled individuals), with a scope of benefits directed primarily toward medical needs during acute illnesses. Thus the provision of LTC services under Medicare is extremely scant. Only limited benefits for skilled nursing home services and home nursing are available; however, benefits are generally much more extensive for hospital care and physician care.

Medicaid, on the other hand, is a welfare program based on criteria of financial indigence. Although the specific eligibility requirements may vary from state to state, the general pattern is that, once the individual has spent down to a certain income, he is eligible for coverage for a variety of medical and socially related services. These include a much broader coverage for LTC than does Medicare, especially for care in nursing homes. The welfare perspective is further maintained under Title XX programs, which may provide additional social service programs to the needy including homemaker day care services or nutritional services. Title XX benefits affecting the elderly vary widely from locality to locality, reflecting the political strength of the aging interest, but, in general, the aged have not received a high proportion of Title XX dollars.

Each of these programs has in common a voucher payment approach which permits government to provide funds either directly to the provider or, in the case of Medicare, to the individual to cover the costs (or part of the charges) of the services included within the benefit package. Although the individual has some choice about who may be selected to provide the services, he cannot elect to spend the money on other activities. Voucher payments used for supplementing other aspects of LTC such as housing subsidies or food stamps are even more direct.

The general reluctance to provide funds directly to the individual as cash payments rather than as some form of voucher can be traced to our historical concept of public responsibility. Although the most equitable way to distribute funds might arguably be to give the individual the money and allow him to purchase whatever he wanted with it, we have not yet evolved a social situation in which we have abrogated public responsibility for the consequences of the individual's actions. Should the individual prefer not to invest in adequate care, society may still find itself responsible for the consequences of that choice. As a check against such an inappropriate investment, we have fallen back on a system of voucher payments where public officials are vested with the responsibility of deciding what set of alternative investments are most effective. In the main, we rely upon professional judgments for such decisions.

More than a lack of trust in the consumer's judgment can be cited on behalf of a purchasing system. As already stated, simple equity in LTC benefits is an insufficient guide because needs vary so greatly. If the government accepts a responsibility to meet individualized needs, it might also be construed as having a responsibility to control access to resources in an individualized manner. In theory a policy of governmental purchase of services as deemed necessary could maximize individual choice within parameters of predetermined needs. Also in theory, services which meet with consumer approval should flourish.

The present system of government purchases for LTC seems only minimally to consult the preferences of the care beneficiaries. The range of consumer choice is often narrow. Depending on geographical area and pressure in services, the benefit available to an individual may be reduced, in practice, to a specific place in a particular nursing home. (This is particularly true because nursing home placements are often arranged from hospitals where cost containment efforts related to federal purchases of acute services create pressures to free the hospital bed.) The line between benefit and coercion is slim under such circumstances. The risk to the proprietors of publicly sponsored nursing homes is minimal (the market is virtually guaranteed), and the risk to the consumer is grave.

As a society, we have not been very creative in looking for solutions to this dilemma. Conceptually, a detailed decision tree could be envisaged in which the individual described the outcomes he sought to maximize and we could then prescribe the most efficient way of achieving those outcomes. Although it is perfectly true that we lack the organized data base to make such judgments at the present time, were this identified as a goal, existing data could be mobilized and a system established which could build upon future experience to improve such decision trees (Kane and Kane 1980). A purchase-of-service system could then be developed with multiple paths rather than one dependent on institutional care. Further, a system with sufficient flexibility could be evolved so that intensive home services could be purchased while an individual waited for an institutional arrangement of his own choice.

In summary, our present public position as a purchaser of services is rather dismal. Huge sums of money are poured into subsidizing institutional care, yet the system has turned out to be inflexible in its ability to meet individualized consumer needs. As later sections will discuss, efforts to ensure the quality of this publicly financed care have also been fraught with problems.

Providing

Although purchase of services predominates in our system, all levels of government are involved in direct provision of LTC services. Governmentally provided services have sprung up piecemeal in response to historical circumstances, leading to inconsistencies in benefits and eligibility.

At the federal level, the Veterans Administration (VA) provides the clearest example of a comprehensive set of publicly provided LTC services directed, in this case, toward those for whom public responsibility is acknowledged because of their prior military service and veteran status. The VA not only supplies pensions and purchases services, but it also operates a comprehensive network of acute and chronic hospitals (including mental hospitals) and residential facilities. With the growing recognition of the "graying" of VA beneficiaries, more LTC programs are being developed, including intensive rehabilitation services, day care, day hospital, home care (with benefits for personal care attendants), and even hospice care. Depending on the regional variations, the VA program in a particular area will evolve into some mixture of directly provided and purchased services.

The VA programs are particularly instructive because they offer the closest analogy in the American context to a national service such as that offered in Great Britain. Despite the artificiality imposed by the fact that the VA provides predominately for men, the VA system provides an opportunity to test the impact of an array of services under single administrative auspices. Genuine choices are permitted to individual beneficiaries, and, because program control is vested in a single organization, it is possible for the various VAs to make modifications in services and to observe their effects.

Other examples of direct service provision are available at the state and local governmental levels. States as well as local governments have operated chronic disease hospitals, and states have had a traditional responsibility for mental hospitals. More recently, joint funding from state and local governments, together with federal funds, has been used for community mental health centers with responsibility for both inpatient and ambulatory services. Although elderly persons should theoretically receive a disproportionate amount of service from such mental health centers (based on incidence of depression and other mental health problems among the elderly), in such age-heterogenous programs the elderly have often received low priority for therapeutic services.

Another age-mixed service program relevant to the elderly is visiting nursing provided through county health departments. Health departments concentrate on both ends of the age spectrum, largely serving case loads of children and elderly. The passage of Medicare gave an impetus to home health programs, and local health departments have been encouraged to form home health agencies—an example of one arm of government acting as payor and another as provider. Homemaker services for patients receiving Medicare-financed home health and for Medicaid patients as means-tested social service provisions are available to a limited extent.

Finally, the network of services sponsored by Area Administration on Aging agencies (AAAs)—what has come to be known as the aging network—must be considered as part of government's direct provision. These include services such as nutritional programs, senior centers, legal aid, and recreational volunteer and employment opportunities for the elderly.

Several points may be made about the provision of direct services in LTC in the United States:

1. The bulk of services directly provided are in the health sector rather than social welfare. The budgets for homemaker assistance, laundry aids, and other community-based social services have lagged behind the direct provision of health services, the payment of health professionals, and the provision of health devices.

2. Although there is precedent for direct provision of chronic hospital and mental hospital services, publicly owned and operated old age homes and residential settings are infrequent.

3. In the health sector, proprietary units have been encouraged and subsidized through government payments (nursing homes and, more recently, home health agencies), whereas there has been much less proprietary development of long-term mental hospitals and hospitals for the retarded, and public provision in these areas is a more acceptable norm. On the other hand, proprietary residential homes and social services have not been particularly encouraged and have not developed to any extent with the exception perhaps of luxury apartment hotels and retirement villas for the affluent and fit elderly.

4. An examination of the publicly provided programs such as VA services, state mental hospitals, AoA programs, and county health department home services reveals a welter of different eligibility criteria, reflecting the differing rationales for the services and different construction of public responsibility and family obligations.

Policing

In its policing role, government is responsible for monitoring the services that it provides or pays for to assure that minimum standards of quality are met. Such standards concern life safety, quality of care, and appropriateness of the use of resources. Institutions have hitherto been the prime targets of official efforts to police LTC.

Quality of care assurance has, for the most part, required that providers adhere to some set of empirically derived structural characteristics that are deemed to be consistent with good care. Such standards have generally been derived from professional "wisdom" rather than empirical exploration or consumer judgment. Typically they have included staff-to-patient ratios, the maintenance of patient records, and professional qualifications of staff. Since the advent of the Medicare and Medicaid programs, the standards that LTC facilities are required to meet in both life safety and quality of care have increased, resulting in the development of nursing homes that have come to resemble hospitals more and more. Some would argue that this upgrading of the technical aspects of care has come at the loss of some of the more homelike qualities that might have been highly desired for at least a portion of the long-term-care residents. Industry spokesmen often depict themselves as hamstrung by regulations.

A number of different policing techniques have been used. These include the licensure of facilities as a prerequisite for their operation; certification of facilities as suitable for participation in federal programs such as Medicare and Medicaid; utilization and appropriateness screening by fiscal intermediaries, carriers, and state agencies; audits for fraud and abuse; and formal reviews of the quality of care through inspection visits such as the medical review program and independent professional review program of Medicaid. More recently, the Professional Standards Review Organization (PSROs) (usually operated in close association with medical societies at the state or local level) have been delegated the responsibility for review of the appropriateness of utilization as well as the quality of care delivered to skilled nursing home patients and, with the agreement of the state, intermediate-care patients as well.

Common to all of these policing activities are a number of problems. While one can readily devise a list of criteria to be met by facilities and even identify deficiencies in performance, it is much more difficult to devise an effective means of dealing with deficiencies once uncovered. Up to the present time, the supply has been less than the demand for these facilities and, as a result, few effective incentives are available. In some states, fines have been levied but remain unpaid. Where facilities have been ordered closed, great problems are created in finding alternative placement, and fears are expressed about the increased mortality that might occur as a result of transferring patients precipitously. Policing is an expensive and touchy business. The cost of assessing, carefully and fully, the performance of facilities is high. And the more thoroughly one conducts such assessments, the closer one comes to interfering by prescribing what a patient should receive.

Perhaps even more critically, mandating a service through quality standards does not ensure that the service is of sufficient quality. For example, standards have been set for the frequency with which physicians should visit their patients in nursing homes. All physician visits, however, are not equivalent. Documentation of physician contact with patient is not synonymous with assuring tht the patient's problems have been carefully studied and that an appropriate therapeutic plan has been developed and monitored. Those engaged in these types of policing activities constantly express the concern that overly zealous regulatory enforcement may drive good providers as well as poor ones from the field.

The monitoring function has been particularly emphasized when government funds services rather than provides them directly. Life safety provisions have been deemed a governmental responsibility in all LTC institutions, regardless of payment source; in this sense, they are analogous to environmental health measures. Quality of care monitoring, on the other hand, has been limited to that care funded by public payment programs. The question of the extent to which funds should be spent in policing care rather than simply delivering it is recurrent. Reactions range from comments that all the money spent in monitoring should be given to the nursing homes to use in patient care, to suggestions that the closest monitoring is an inadequate substitution for removing care from the proprietary sector.

Publicly provided services also require policing, a fact not well appreciated. It is reasonable to assume that the elaborate quality assurance mechanisms arose in the United States to regulate the private entrepreneur. In Great Britain, where publicly provided health and social services are the norm, monitoring is notably underdeveloped. If decisions are made to move more extensively into providing direct public LTC services, whether in institutions, congregate living facilities, or the community, some method of ensuring their quality must be developed.

The proper policing of publicly provided services is worthy of further consideration and study. Perhaps it is unreasonable to expect that providers can police their own activities; this is reminiscent of the child guarding the cookie jar. The models available for examining quality control in the publicly provided services are not auspicious. Centralized systems such as the Veterans Administration or the Public Health Service have central office personnel who are responsible for promulgating and enforcing standards, but rarely are such personnel close enough to the scene to get their own factual information. Autonomous review bodies within an organization (for example, police review boards) tend to be subject to charges of self-interest. Perhaps when services are largely publicly provided, voluntary watchdog organizations are necessary to monitor quality of care just as public monitoring is necessary to oversee the activities of voluntary and proprietary care givers.

Policing for community-based LTC and, more particularly, the social service components presents an enormous problem. Home-based services are not as amenable to monitoring as hospital care because of (1) the multiplicity of delivery sites, and (2) the comparative lack of control over variables of service when the provider is a guest in the recipient's home. The skills of the homemaker, the geriatric visitor, or the social worker have a high component of "art" as opposed to technology, and art of care does not lend itself readily to standards setting. The difficulty in mounting quality control over community-based programs is a major basis for public reluctance to support such care. One solution may lie in greater reliance on the consumer to assess the usefulness of the services he receives.

Consumer feedback can drive the quality of care only under proper conditions: (1) the consumer must have genuine choices, (2) the consumer must have a vehicle to express feedback, (3) the consumer must not be subject to reprisals when negative feedback is given, and (4) the consumer must understand the requirements of an adequate service. The first three conditions are rarely met in institutional long-term care and may pose problems in any publicly delivered or funded community-based program. In the institutional example, the consumer is typically "placed" in an available nursing home bed with little initial choice. The mixture of isolation, frailty, and dependence on the caretaker makes any negative feedback unlikely. If the elderly institutional resident were to decide to act, no clear mechanisms would be available. Rarely does the recipient of care wield the LTC payment dollars. Satisfaction of his complaints is not timely, and meanwhile he may be placed in double jeopardy because of them.

Community-based services may have the same problem, although in less dramatic form. Certainly an individual has more control over access to his own home than to an institution. Nevertheless, the clients are often vulnerable and their complaints are less irrelevant if the choice is whether to buy a specific service (meals, home health, homemaking) or do without it. The last condition of effective consumer feedback—that the consumer understand the nature of an adequate service—is also hard to meet in community-based long-term care. Here much of the necessary job is educational. An example is the exploitation of the elderly by unscrupulous door-to-door hearing aid vendors (Powers 1974, 1976). One method of handling the problem is by developing standards for reimbursement. Even assuming that definitions could be reached, however, the elderly consumer would be the ultimate out-of-pocket victim. Another method of redress is legislative, prohibiting various business practices and requiring licensure for hearing aid vendors. A more basic remedy is education of the potential consumer, a process that needs to start well before old age. This one example of hearing aid services can be multiplied many times to include the large range of services that are part of long-term care.

Changes in service provision or payment for service necessitate considering new forms of policing. If our public policy is to develop a large network of community-based social services, we would be irresponsible not to monitor their quality. If, in another example, a case management system is developed to make matches between needs and resources, its caseworkers must also be subject to monitoring. The responsibility of acting as gatekeeper to services is onerous and the technology indeterminant. The policing function, therefore, must also be supplemented by other strategies, discussed below, such as consumer protection, prevention, and promotion of informed consumers.

Protecting

A number of public agencies have the responsibility for protecting the rights and entitlements of the individual. In the most clear-cut situations, when individuals are deemed to be incapable of making decisions for themselves, public guardianship can be instituted. Under such provisions, the public agency serves as a legal guardian for the individual, acting in his behalf.

This public role is fraught with complexity, particularly when the expressed interests of the LTC recipients and their families diverge. Public guardianship or declarations of incompetence may serve family interests most. At the worst end of the spectrum of motives is financial gain and, at the best, an earnest desire to protect an elderly relative from accident or harm. On the other hand, some family caretakers themselves need protection from intolerable burdens. This is true of elderly relatives who are in poor health. It is argued, too, that it is patently unfair to fetter the early retirement years of a fit elderly person with the care of a more debilitated parent. Both parties to the equation are vulnerable: the LTC recipient because of functional limitations and the relative because of guilt. Documented physical abuse of elderly persons (granny bashing) is on the rise in England and might become more prevalent in the United States with increasing community care of the very infirm.

The need for protection of the elderly should be conceptualized in a way that distinguishes between physical frailty, requiring a guarantee of a person's rights to make decisions, and mental frailty. Moreover, the extent to which a person should be protected, either at home or in institutions, is problematic. Protecting the mentally disoriented against wandering may not be worthwhile if physical restraints are required. Perhaps in a nursing home that is really a home, falls should be almost as frequent as in the community. There is also a danger that, once social services are involved, old people will be urged into institutions in order to eliminate risks that were part of a lifelong environment.

At a more general level, the rights of elderly consumers of LTC in institutions are judged to be an appropriate concern of authorities like the Federal Trade Commission (Taylor 1979). Here the efforts are directed toward protecting the consumer against various forms of fraud by assuring that the client is fully informed about the procedures being carried out by the LTC institution; that adequate safeguards have been made for handling such things as personal funds; and that no contract is entered into without the consumer's being fully aware of its consequences. Ironically, in a reversal of the expression of the policing role, the FTC provisions seem to extend only toward patients who do not utilize federal funds. Once the federal government becomes a third-party payor for the care of LTC patients, the jurisdiction returns to the agency responsible for the payment.

Other areas of protection have not been so well articulated by current programs. Such tasks as clarifying the right to treatment have not been identified as the particular responsibility of any federal agency. Patients dependent on third-party federal programs, for example, are routinely discriminated against by providers; although health care has been deemed a right, it is not at all clear how the rights of the consumer are interfaced with the rights of the provider to refuse to provide services if he is not satisfied with the payment or the payment mechanism. Similarly, we have not yet developed any clarity about public responsibility to persons demanding the right to die.

Preventing

The relationship of prevention to the provision of long-term care has been frequently discussed. Advocates of preventive services suggest that investments in early stages might prevent the need for LTC or minimize its extent and duration. Public responsibility for engaging in such preventive activities can be based on a number of arguments. The first rests upon evidence of efficiency, namely, that an investment at an early stage would be more efficient than supporting the consequences of the problem later on. A second argument is based on the assumption that preventive measures can alleviate unnecessary suffering.

A number of programs have been proposed and developed to work with populations while they are still independent and intact in the hopes of warding off functional and social disability. Under such a heading would come the provision of recreational services, bereavement counseling, screening programs, and other forms of active case finding. Unfortunately, the data to establish the efficacy of prevention are extremely scant. The dilemma faced is the high aggregate cost of any preventive activity, owing to the large number of individuals eligible compared with the number whose natural course would otherwise have been different. At the present time, insufficient data exist to support any decision for or against heavy investment in that preventive area. There are, however, and will continue to be strong pressures for the development of such services. To the extent that public agencies choose to provide or to pay for such services, they have the potential to stimulate large areas of services which will demand resources that might be expended in other areas of long-term care.

Paradoxically, an important aspect of prevention concerns the management of acute problems, including tertiary care. This seeming contradiction comes about because the elderly are particularly vulnerable to iatrogenic complications. A month in the hospital can leave an older person in reduced functional status as a result of inactivity, lack of stimulation, and the passiveness of the patient role. A range of programs are possible to prevent such deterioration. In addition, prompt and complete diagnosis and treatment of treatable conditions can prevent a spiraling cycle of interrelated disabilities.

Because public responsibility for acute care of the elderly is largely separated from the LTC component, anomalous situations arise. Probably the single most important event that policymakers would like to prevent (or postpone) is institutionalization. If so, the public policies for providing acute care seem poorly designed to achieve that end. The policing function for the acute sector demands rapid discharge. Without data, one nevertheless suspects that false economies occur. A week saved in an acute hospital can lead to a lifetime in an LTC facility, and some individuals would be able to remain in the community if time were available to work out the arrangements.

Thus, the hospital physicians are judged by their economies in the hospital sector and many tend to overprescribe nursing homes. More and better efforts are needed to effect earlier discharge planning from hospitals. Several options can be considered from earlier involvement of appropriate ancillary staff to allow adequate time for identification and exploration of alternatives, to the establishment of special units, e.g., Geriatric Evaluation Units, where more thorough assessments of patients could be conducted. Such assessments have led to substantial shifts in patient dispositions (Williams, et al., 1973; Brocklehurst 1978).

Furthermore, Medicare as a public policy statement militates against having a person return home for a period of community care on a trial basis; if it later materializes that an institutional placement is necessary, Medicare benefits cannot be collected without an intervening rehospitalization. The isolation of LTC from medical care provision and the factors discussed above have helped create the inexorable sequence of hospital to nursing home. Although those articulating goals for LTC are desirous of preventing institutionalization, for those at the hospital level it is not a primary concern. Perhaps PSRO preadmission review of those referred to nursing homes from hospitals could help bridge the gap. This seems unlikely, however, because the PSRO role has been confined to certifying that the given applicant meets the definition of a person requiring a particular level of LTC, and because PSROs are even more strongly accountable for unnecessary days spent in acute hospitals.

Of course, the prevention of deterioration in functional status and of institutionalization also depends on a range of community LTC services that are not readily available. High on the list is home help; also valuable are shopping services, transportation, home improvements and modifications, night sitting, laundry services, incontinence aids, meals on wheels, and day centers (where, in addition to socialization, such services as baths are available for those who do not have access to a suitable tub, as well as podiatry, hairdressing, and perhaps even physical therapy). Specially designed housing units that combine privacy for the individual or family group with opportunities for congregate meals when desired and emergency access to a caring person could eliminate the need for institutional care for a substantial segment of people.

In England such housing (called sheltered housing) was designed for persons with moderate needs for LTC; however, experience has shown that persons who have deteriorated in functional status when in sheltered housing have generally been contained in that environment rather than removed to an institution. Community services such as those listed above must also be available to sheltered housing residents to enable them to remain in that status with increasing immobility, incontinence, or some confusion. The preventive impact of sheltered housing is felt only if vacancies are available before an institutional solution is taken; in England, tremendous queues occur for sheltered housing, and waits of six months to a year are not uncommon. If sheltered housing is to become a planned service designed to maximinze autonomy and quality of life, an adequate number of such units must be developed, along with the services that will enable a person to wait in the community until sheltered housing becomes available.

An American analogue of sheltered housing is the shared dwelling arrangements that have sprung up around the country. Often under voluntary agency auspices, such programs arrange for mutually compatible elderly persons to share houses and apartments. Sometimes the sponsoring agency owns or rents the dwellings and provides staff; in other arrangements, the sponsor may be acting only as an intermediary. At this point, descriptions of house sharing are more common in the daily newspaper than in the professional literature. They may represent a practical and creative approach that redistributes housing and companionship with minimal front-end costs.

Peopling

Professional personnel.—The provision of long-term-care services is generally accepted to be extremely manpower intensive. A wide variety of personnel are involved, and new career pathways seem to emerge daily. Government roles in the area of peopling seem to extend from exerting influence on the educational and training mechanisms to produce different numbers and types of LTC personnel, to providing direct incentives to individuals to pursue careers in LTC-related fields. In some cases the government may be the direct employer of such individuals, using such personnel for its own programs of direct-service provision or assigning these individuals to other agencies for this purpose. In other cases, it may simply set standards for training, encourage the development of curriculum materials, mandate educational requirements for licensure and certification of professionals, or require some level of continued training.

Before a rational public policy can be formulated regarding manpower, data are required about the kinds of personnel actually needed. Considerable overlap already exists among the functions and skills of various LTC providers, suggesting some interchangeability. Furthermore, new categories of personnel could be encouraged into the LTC arena, if a need for them is defined. Both vertical and horizontal substitutions are possible. The former is usually envisaged as cost saving; for example, nurse practitioners might be able to perform some of the functions of physicians, and nurses' aides might be able to perform some nursing functions. It would also be possible to promote vertical substitution in a more expensive direction; for instance, a concerted effort could be made to upgrade nursing home social workers by requiring MSW credentials. Horizontal substitution involves change across professions; for example, social workers rather than nurses in charge of LTC institutions, occupational therapists instead of social workers leading therapeutic groups, nurses instead of social workers making social assessments and referring individuals to community resources.

Horizontal substitution on a grand scale might not have any economic implications for program cost but rather grow out of an effort to change the very nature of service delivery. Although newly sensitized manpower may be needed, such a goal is not dependent on production of newly trained geriatric specialists but on redirecting the energies and abilities of those who have already received basic professional education. On the other hand, a kind of substitution where one discipline deliberately takes on some of the attributes of another could be cost effective. The health visitor in England is a district nurse who has had added training in social work; interestingly, however, health visitors have replaced neither district nurses nor district social workers, but have instead developed a separate role on the team.

Evolving a strategy for professional manpower development is necessarily complicated. As indicated above, new manpower is not always an answer. Sometimes no absolute shortages exist, yet the elderly do not receive the benefit of the most advanced knowledge and skills. Medical care is an interesting case in point. The typical physician in primary care (general practitioners and internists) see a preponderance of persons over age 65 in their practices and so, too, do the majority of medical and surgical subspecialists. The need seems to be one of redirection of such personnel to consider the special requirements of the elderly. On the other hand, geriatric specialists are required for teaching, consultation, and practice in specialized geriatric settings, and the infusion of geriatric content through the whole medical practice probably requires the production of some specialists. Considering all these factors and the possibility of some substitutability, Kane and his colleagues (1981) conservatively estimated that 8,000 geriatric medical specialists would be required by 1990 and suggested ways that this controlled growth could be stimulated through public policy.

Historically, heavy governmental investment has been made at federal and state levels in the basic preparation and continuing education of professional groups involved in delivering LTC. The public investment in medical education, nursing education, and social work education has been substantial, but, until recently, there has been little targeting toward LTC, either toward development of geriatric subspecialists in a particular profession or toward sponsoring trainees with obligations to become involved in LTC. Lately, some deliberate efforts have been made to stimulate development of manpower especially qualified for LTC. Policies have not been consistent, however; as a case in point, federal funds are used to support the training of geriatric nurse practitioners, but such practitioners working without direct supervision are specifically ineligible for reimbursement under the Medicare program.

The dilemma of the geriatric nurse practitioner whose skills have no ready market raises questions about the extent to which the government should advocate or mandate the use of preferred types of providers. Where data exist to show that quality of service is equivalent, the insistence on one type of provider over another may be counterproductive. In most instances, overly restrictive regulations based on some assumed set of qualitative effects or pursued in an attempt to save money by relying on less expensive personnel may lead to unforeseen complications. Federal initiatives have adversely affected nurse practitioner utilization, despite studies showing that nurse practitioners can provide high-quality primary care for nursing home patients (Kane, et al., 1976) and elderly persons living in the community (Master, et al., 1980). Medicare's refusal to pay for such care without on-site physician supervision has rendered the use of such sorely needed personnel infeasible.

The history of federal intervention in the development of manpower programs has been fraught with repeated vacillation between conditions of undersupply and oversupply because of the lack of adequate data to forecast market needs (GMENAC 1979). An important question is the extent to which the government should exercise some interpretive judgment on reading manpower projections produced by interested professional groups who extrapolate the status quo into the future. The government has the choice of a passive manpower policy or a rather active one that creates and eliminates manpower categories through training and payment incentives. The style adopted largely reflects social values.

Nonprofessional personnel.—So far we have discussed the education and stimulation of professional personnel. LTC, however, requires a large labor force that may not need advanced training to any large extent. What they do need is an enjoyment of people, regardless of age; compassion; common sense; and a willingness to perform a variety of tasks as they might be needed rather than a rote reliance on job descriptions. Such persons could be functioning as care assistants (better terminology than nurses' aides) in residential facilities, as home helps, or as home health assistants. Our largest nonprofessional LTC work force is presently in nursing homes where the turnover of personnel is notoriously high.

Recognizing the lack of preparation of many nurses' aides, some states have developed regulations for continuing education of nursing home personnel. Although the educational route to job upgrading is the familiar one, it may not be the correct solution here. Indeed, in states where nursing homes are mandated to fund training for aides in their employ more than a year, anecdotal evidence suggests a prevalent practice of terminating the employee just before the investment in education would be necessary. If such is the case, a public policy regarding peopling has boomeranged.

The real reasons for the lack of an adequate nonprofessional work force probably have little to do with educational preparation but are linked more to salary, job conditions, and expectations. In many English communities, home helps recruited by the municipality are deliberately paid slightly more than could be realized by domestic work in the private sector. Care assistants in residential facilities have been known to move up the career ladder in residential care, even to the point of deputy director or facility director.

Personnel selection is a paramount consideration. A disadvantage of a purchase system as opposed to direct provision is that the payor cannot assume that private individuals will have selection criteria that emphasize caring attributes. Similarly, home helps and care attendants require an administrative support system on which they can count; in the case of the home help, it goes without saying that she must be guaranteed a continued source of work and cannot be paid on a job basis. If a given home help is hired for three days a week, she must be guaranteed a job on those days.

Stereotyped ideas about who would be willing to perform nonprofessional LTC functions are also counterproductive and perhaps reflect the professional devaluing of actual concrete service. Because such jobs can be flexibly arranged as part-time or odd-hour jobs and because of their humanitarian appeal, they can (and, in England, do) attract a range of persons, even housewives with professional education in nonhealth fields.

For jobs to have intrinsic satisfaction, they must be conceptualized as more than menial and routine. Indeed, a sense of judgment must be cultivated in care assistants in and out of institutions; they must know where to give priority, how to consult the wishes of the elderly person, when *not* to do something (in order to foster independence), when sitting and talking to a client (or his family) are more important than cleaning the floor, or when it would be better for a home help to spend an hour walking to the grocery store with an elderly person than cleaning the kitchen.

Whether government initiatives can stimulate the development of a cadre of intelligent and committed nonprofessional workers in a proprietary system of care is unclear. Certainly isolated instances of model staffing can be cited in the United States; for example, one nursing home in Colorado decided to change all nursing aides to care assistants and expected a mixture of counseling, patient care planning, physical nursing, and advocacy as the job description (Kane, et al., 1979*b*). The articulated goal was to encourage the independent functioning and well-being of the patient and even to promote discharge when possible. According to the administrator, this job was attractive to newly graduated college students in social sciences (with no previous practical nursing experience) as well as to long-time nurses' aides, and very little turnover occurred over a three-year period. It would be unrealistic, however, to expect such attitudes to be reflected across the whole private sector. We might be a little more optimistic that a program of public social services, both institutional and noninstitutional, could economically centralize efforts to recruit, select, and motivate a nonprofessional staff.

Promoting

Many of the activities already described might be identified with different types of goals. There is a need, however, to distinguish between process and outcomes. An important part of public policy is to improve the public's ability to articulate what it seeks to achieve through its policies. Here we move from pursuing goals on the basis of fixed ideologies to that of increasing the state of public knowledge about a situation. Examples of this type of public policy might include educational efforts designed to change public attitudes about aging through programs aimed at the professional (e.g., health professionals), those aimed at the public in general through the use of the mass media, and perhaps those aimed at the elderly themselves. The last example might include promotion of more informed consumers who are aware of the options available to them and the services to which they are entitled. A second level of promotion would include the development of adequate knowledge on which to base future programs. This would include support of both research and demonstration efforts including the careful analysis of programs already conducted.

Policymaking/Priority Setting and Planning

In many ways the foregoing tasks involve the development of programs designed to maximize certain outcomes while avoiding untoward consequences. It is only when the goals are clearly in mind that one can choose among a number of available strategies. For example, decisions about the scope of benefits and level of eligibility for the various types of long-term-care services including home health care, homemaking services, day care, and sheltered housing will have profound effects on the ways in which these services are given and received. Despite the often-expressed fears of too much government regulation, there appears to be strong support for a major public role in LTC planning, to anticipate the effects of such policies and initiating these programs deliberately. The heavy investment of public funds in these areas mandates such an approach. The concerns, however, are equally strong that such programs not usurp the role now being played by private resources, both formal and informal. If a goal of increased client autonomy and concomitant emphasis on community-based care is pursued (and we hope it will be), it will be essential that some means of limiting the flow of resources into institutions (i.e., nursing homes) be established. Without such a constraint, we despair of seeing any significant degree of community care.

Calling for a cutback before an alternative is in place is bound to produce opposition. There is, within the federal government, a substantial difference of opinion as to how much data need be amassed before definitive steps are begun to shift the locus of care. In its report on the undesirable effects of Medicaid funding of nursing home care, the Comptroller General (1979) has argued that sufficient evidence is now available to allow us to move boldly ahead with a community-oriented program. In the letter published as an appendix to that report, HEW urges a more cautious path with a series of demonstration projects prior to shifting national policy on a grand scale. The question is not simply whether alternatives to the nursing home can provide equal or better care, but to whom such services should be offered. If publicly funded alternatives are more appealing and accessible, they may be most attractive to those now relying on private informal support. The increased utilization may well represent meeting a previously unserved need but at a high aggregate cost (Kane and Kane 1980). A better assessment technology is needed to define levels and types of need (Kane and Kane 1981), and a more thoughtful policy is required to set priorities about which target groups we seek to reach, with what consequences.

Moreover, if community care is an agreed-upon goal, the organizational responsibility for public implementation is open to debate. From a logical perspective, one can argue that such care should be viewed as a social, rather than a medical, service. Such designation, however, has major implications for both the form of care rendered and the size of the resource pool available to support it.

Important policy issues revolve around the question of what balance should be struck between public and private services through either their direct provision or purchase. Should public investments be made on the basis of the estimates of probable yield? To what extent can investments be made in individuals who are deemed to be high risk?

Because the role of the public agencies is so ubiquitous with regard to long-term care, any decision in one segment is likely to have strong repercussions in many others. For example, the imposition of stringent regulations with regard to life safety codes or the imposition of strong certificate-of-need limitations on the creation of new nursing home beds will affect the size and the shape of the nursing home resource pool. Decisions about methods of payment for long-term care will provoke profound responses in terms of the available resources.

Within the realm of planning, much of the burden falls on the Health Systems Agencies (HSAs), which are responsible for developing a more rational approach for assessing and meeting the needs for health services. Because this program is grounded in the health services system, rather than the social services, an obvious danger is that its actions will be weighted toward health care; if so, the danger is that the HSA will perpetuate the medical model by focusing on the appropriate level of nursing home needed. On the other hand, a less obvious, but very real, risk is that the HSA will dismiss the problem as social and ignore the whole field, despite its obvious relevance to health.

The HSA has a very direct role in shaping the LTC system through its use of Certificate of Need (CON). The power to authorize or to deny development of different sections of the LTC industry will directly affect the supply of resources. To the extent that a larger supply of LTC choices represents market competition, the HSA determines the degree of such competition. However, because supply is also tied to utilization, limits on growth are seen as the only way to halt increasing use of nursing homes and possibly other forms of LTC as well. The HSA, as a planning body, faces a dilemma—the need to weigh increased consumer choice against the risk of increasing the total costs of care.

It seems inevitable that the need and/or demand for LTC will continue to exceed greatly the resources available. Priorities will have to be set on the basis of one or more rationing policies. These could include: limiting services to those who ask; limiting the number of services made available to any single individual; providing incentives for and developing expectations for family responsibility; queuing on a first-come-first-served basis; or queuing with a central case management or triaging system to ensure that the greatest needs are met the quickest. In a planned system with well-publicized benefits, some queuing would seem necessary, even if the entitlements were quite limited. If choice is also to be offered to the individual within a system of scarce resources, the problems are exacerbated.

It is clear that each of these approaches to delimiting services comes at a cost. There is an apparent inconsistency between meeting the demands of only those able to articulate their needs and providing a service as an entitlement to all citizens. Public responsibility has generally been interpreted to mean some major role in seeking out persons in need. At the same time, any program of vigorous government assumption of responsibility runs the risk of fostering increased dependence. Past welfare programs have been accused of creating perverse results by just this type of dependency breeding.

Restricting the number of services available to any single individual runs counter to a policy of trying to meet the varying needs of people who may be afflicted through no fault of their own. Past welfare programs have been established on the basis of a minimum benefit package, but such programs have been accused of being inequitable. In some cases this inequity has been successfully challenged in the law courts. The final decision on this approach may rest with the issue of how high that minimum is set. To the extent that certain services are covered and others not, there is a differential stimulation of the long-term-care industry. For example, the Medicare program has been criticized for its heavy support of the hospital at the cost of neglecting potentially less expensive primary care. Unfortunately, services which are available at a lower unit cost are often demanded in a much higher volume so that the overall savings are less obvious.

The role of the family in assuming some responsibility along with the public continues to be a perplexing one. At the one extreme, we seek programs which will encourage families to continue providing services to the level of their capacity. As a society, however, we are not prone to incur family disruption as a cost of providing long-term care. Nor have we, even implicitly, determined the degree to which we are willing to sacrifice one generation for another. If we have not resolved the extent to which we are willing, on a societal basis, to expend funds on behalf of the elderly at the risk of decreasing the resources available for the education of the young, we are even less clear as to how to handle the resource allocation problem at the family unit level.

Nor should the family issue be articulated solely as a decision about the extent to which relatives should be relieved of responsibility by public policy. It is clearly possible that some community services to the elderly could strengthen family ties and improve the quality and quantity of interaction in families across generations. When families are asked to share the responsibility in the knowledge that outside support and respite care are available, they may be more able to muster partial support and do so without the resentment that would cloud relationships. Research is needed to determine systematically the effects of various supportive programs on family involvement.

General Issues
Long-Term Care and Death

Pundits say that the best way to ensure a long life is to "get a chronic illness and take good care of it." The converse of this statement is the truism that all long-term care ends in death. The nature of public responsibility for the dying elderly person has been long ignored. Because the topic has been neglected, very little information is available about how and where elderly people die; we suspect that many die in unfamiliar circumstances, alone in a crowded hospital, or in an ambulance being hastily rushed away from home or a long-term-care facility.

Over the past 15 years, the national interest in "death and dying" has taken on elements of a social movement (Cohen 1979; Halper 1979). The pressures directed toward achieving a more humane and dignified way of death have found expression in new institutions—hospices—to enhance the physical and psychological comfort of the dying. For the most part, the hospice serves cancer patients; the prototypical recipient of hospice care is the person who has a terminal illness with a predictable short course (measured in week or months). Although figures are not easily available, the modal age of the hospice patient is thought to be over 65.

In response to pressures from the hospice movement, policymakers are now evaluating the extent to which hospice benefits should be covered through funded programs. Ironically, however, any reforms in care of the dying introduced through this ferment are likely to have little impact on the bulk of long-term-care patients. The major principles of hospice, including a commitment to palliative care and to holistic treatment of the dying as living persons, should be applicable to persons in either community-based or institution-based long-term care. Nobody has proposed, however, that even the LTC patients who develop terminal cancer should be transferred to a hospice environment for the rest of their care. Such a practice would immediately swamp the system. The consideration of hospice raises many value questions. Is society more willing to make a large investment in the quality of dying of a relatively small number of persons than in the quality of living of a larger number? Can hospice-type care be generalized so that its essential characteristics can be applied at the terminal stage to any long-term-care recipient?

Care of the dying combines all the roles we described in the previous section. As payor, the public might want to consider an expanded range of benefits. As provider, the public might wish to organize a service that would prevent the elderly from dying friendless and alone; volunteers might play an important role in such a program. Housing programs will need to take into account whether a person could live and die in the planned units. As policer, the monitoring agencies might consider developing standards for when an individual should be transferred from a long-term-care facility to die. A study of the PSRO's record in long-term care (Kane, et al., 1979a) showed that this was one area untouched by utilization review committees. Peopling is also relevant; a cadre of care givers must be trained who are able to give humane care to the dying. Although few suggest solutions, many authorities agree that a responsible long-term-care program must develop a stance toward death. In the words of a British geriatrician:

> Though much regarding death will involve ethical consideration, nonetheless very practical points arise from the structuring of a care programme. The attitudes to and management of the dying will affect the attitudes to and management of the living prior to it. No organized long-term care program can ignore it. It is the second most important event in a person's life. In my opinion, there is nothing worse than arranging a long-term care programme and then having to transfer a patient to strange surroundings and institutions to die. [Foote, 1980]

Unresolved Dilemmas

Suppose that there were public agreement that the valued objectives in long-term care are maximization of independent physical and social functioning and personal choice within a community setting whenever possible and within residential institutional settings when necessary. Many questions would arise about the extent to which the public should foster these goals, the extent of family responsibility, the level of government that should be involved, and the mix of public roles that should be employed to achieve that end. Some of the consideration of means would be fiscal and political, and some would also involve values and beliefs (for instance, in local versus centralized authority or in free enterprise versus government provision). Nevertheless, the ultimate goal would be clear, and some of the questions about means would be amenable to research so that some values could be exchanged for facts. For example, the belief in the importance of a primary care physician might change if research showed that functional status diminished in individuals cared for by a physician as opposed to a geriatric nurse practitioner.

Again, assuming commitment to an overall goal that can be stated in roughly measurable terms, some strategic considerations arise when articulation of public policy involves trade-offs among cherished principles. For example, equity in provision of services is gained at the expense of individualized plans; local community responsibility and decentralization increase the likelihood that an overall plan is responsive to the needs of a given area but decrease ability to guarantee equity.

Throughout this paper we have made many allusions to the experience in Great Britain. Indeed, the British system shows more commitment to community and to an array of practical LTC services than does our own. It is important to note, however, that Britain is a much more homogeneous society than is the United States, with much less history of inequities in governmental provisions. It is also geographically much more compact. Despite these advantages, the British system of LTC is still geographically based, and regional differences in population mix, migratory habits, available work force, culture, and other factors have required a different mix of LTC services, even in counties 20 miles apart.

Diversity is obviously much greater across the United States. Some regional decision-making responsibility about the nature of LTC provisions would seem to be necessary within statutory limitations that mandated a range of services and within a value commitment to basic goals. The fear in the United States, of course, is that the price of regionalization will be inequities and, in some geographic areas, neglect of the elderly. Unless the decision-making and planning units are fairly small, however, the responsibility is diffused and the problems and conditions of the elderly needing LTC become less visible. A large state is much too large an area for meaningful local planning. The infusion of local citizens in the planning and management process (analogous to local public involvement in schools) would go a long way to familiarize people with the issues and the real conditions. Some of the abuses and neglect in LTC occur because the problems are removed from the view of ordinary citizens who are concerned about their communities.

Much earlier we made the point that long-term-care policy is often discussed in the context of the institution. The merits of community-based care are constantly debated, and many public experiments had their genesis in an effort to determine whether alternatives to nursing home care were feasible and affordable. To some extent, the focus on the dichotomy between institution and community places too much attention on locus of service rather than its nature. It is possible to envisage a congregate living situation that provides the necessary physical, emotional, and social care while maintaining privacy, dignity, and choice for individuals. In some instances, congregate living might be the preferred situation because of its opportunity for some social interaction and stimulation that might not be available to a very frail person living alone without access to relatives or friends. Both institution and community will, we hope, change in the future so that their features become more blended; not only should we expect much more care and service brought to the home, but we should also expect more residential facilities that take on the characteristics of home.

We began this paper with a discussion of the importance of values and beliefs in forging a concept of public responsibility. In much of the remainder we have touched upon the many interrelated roles that could be played by governments in implementing an LTC policy. For each of the public roles—pensioning, purchasing, providing, policing, protecting, preventing, peopling, promoting, and policymaking/priority setting and planning—the decisions about what should be offered become a matter of collective value judgment. Commitment to goals such as community long-term care; autonomy and choice for elderly citizens requiring LTC; dignified life conditions; and least restrictive care provision (implying minimized management through drugs and restraints) must precede the development of the services to support those goals. Soon enough it will be apparent that the achievement of the goal is necessarily imperfect and that rationing of services will be required, but without widely shared initial value commitments, it is unlikely that steps will be taken in the right directions. Without being categorical, we personally favor the value of autonomy over safety, and of dignified life over prolonging life as long as scientifically possible, although others might place a higher value on safety and on risk avoidance for elderly persons in need of LTC. The worst conceptual error, in our opinion, is to ignore the fact that safety and life preservation are sometimes at odds with independence, personal choice, and human dignity. If we strive to develop a policy with all good outcomes, there is a danger of achieving none.

References

Beattie, W. M., Jr. "Aging and the Social Services," in *Handbook of Aging and the Social Sciences*, ed. R. H. Binstock and E. Shanas. New York: Van Nostrand Reinhold, 1976.
Binstock, R. H., and Levin, M. A. "The Political Dilemmas of Intervention Policies," in *Handbook of Aging and the Social Sciences*, ed. R. H. Binstock and E. Shanas. New York: Van Nostrand Reinhold, 1976.

116   Kane and Kane

Birnbaum, H. *A National Profile of Catastrophic Illness.* DHEW Publ # (PHS) 78-3201, Hyattsville, Md.: National Center for Health Services Research, 1978.
Brocklehust, J. D.; Carthy, M. H.; Leeming, J. T.; and Robinson, J. M. "Medical Screening of Old People Accepted for Residential Care." *Lancet* 1978, pp. 141–43.
Brody, E. M. "Aging of the Family." *Annals of the American Academy of Political Social Science* 438 (1978): 13–27.
Callahan, D. "Health and Society: Some Ethical Imperatives," in *Doing Better and Feeling Worse,* ed. J. Knowles. New York: W. W. Norton, 1977.
Cohen, K. P. *Hospice: Prescription for Terminal Care.* Germantown, Md.: Aspen Systems, 1979.
Community Council of Greater New York. *Dependency in the Elderly of New York City: Policy and Service Implications of the U.S.–U.K. Cross-National Geriatric Community.* Study Report of a Research Utilization Workshop held on March 23, 1978, New York, Community Council of Greater New York, 1978.
Eggert, G., et al. *Community-Based Care for the Long-Term Patient.* Waltham, Mass.: Levinson Policy Institute, 1975.
Estes, C. L. *The Aging Enterprise: A Critical Examination of Social Policies and Services for the Aged.* San Francisco, Calif.: Jossey-Bass, 1979.
Flanagan, J. "A Research Approach to Improving Our Quality of Life." *American Psychology* 33 (1978): 138–47.
Foote, C. K. A., personal communication, 1980.
Gibson, R. M., and Fisher, C. R. "Age Differences in Health Care Spending, Fiscal Year 1977." *Social Security Bulletin* 42 (1979): 3–16.
Graduate Medical Education National Advisory Committee (GMENAC). *Interim Report to the Secretary* (DHEW Publ #HRA 79-633). Washington, D.C.: G.P.O., 1979.
Grauer, H., and Birnbom, F. "A Geriatric Functional Rating Scale to Determine the Need for Institutional Care." *Journal of the American Geriatrics Society* 20 (1975): 472–76.
Halper, T. "On Death, Dying and Terminality: Today, Yesterday and Tomorrow." *Journal of Health Politics, Policy and Law* 4 (1979): 11–29.
Harris, Louis, and Associates. *Myth and Reality of Aging in America.* Washington, D.C.: National Council on Aging, 1975.
Hasenfeld, I., and English, R. A. "Human Service Organizations: A Conceptual Overview," in *Human Service Organizations,* ed. I. Hasenfeld and R. A. English. Ann Arbor: University of Michigan Press, 1974.
Hill, R. "Decision Making and the Family Life Cycle," in *Social Structure and the Family: Generational Relationships,* ed. E. Shanas and G. F. Streib, Englewood Cliffs, N.J.: Prentice Hall, 1963.
Hudson, R. B. "Political and Budgetary Consequences of an Aging Population." *National Journal* 10 (1978): 1699–1705.
Isaacs, B., and Neville, Y. *The Measurement of Need in Old People.* Scottish Health Service Studies #34. Perth, Scotland: Milne, Tannahill & Methven, 1975.
Isaacs, B., and Neville, Y. "The Interval as a Method of Measurement." *British Journal of Prevention and Social Medicine* 30 (1976): 79–85.
Kane, R. L.; Jorgensen, L. A.; Teteberg, B.; and Kuwahara, J. "Is Good Nursing Home Care Feasible?" *JAMA* 235 (1976): 516–19.
Kane, R. L., and Kane, R. A. "Alternatives to Institutional Care of the Elderly: Beyond the Dichotomy." *The Gerontologist* 20 (1980): 249–59.
Kane, R. A., and Kane, R. L. *Assessing the Elderly: A Practical Guide to Measurement.* Lexington, Mass.: D. C. Heath, 1981.
Kane, R. A.; Kane, R. L.; Kleffel, D.; Brook, R. H.; Eby, C.; and Goldberg, G. A. *The PSRO and the Nursing Home.* Vol. 2: *Ten Demonstration Projects in PSRO Long-Term Care Review.* R-2459/2-HCFA. Santa Monica, Calif.: The Rand Corporation, 1979b.

Kane, R. A.; Kane, R. L.; Kleffel, D.; Brook, R. H.; Eby, C.; Goldberg, G. A.; Rubenstein, L. Z.; and VanRyzin, J. *The PSRO and the Nursing Home.* Vol. 1: *An Assessment of PSRO Long-Term Care Review.* R-2549/1-HCFA. Santa Monica, Calif.: The Rand Corporation, 1979*a.*

Kane, R. L.; Solomon, D. H.; Beck, J. C.; Keeler, E.; and Kane, R. A. *Geriatrics in the United States: Manpower Projections and Training Considerations.* Lexington, Mass.: D. C. Heath, 1981.

Levy, C. *Social Work Ethics.* New York: Human Sciences Press, 1976.

Master, R. J.; Feltin, M.; Jainchill, J.; Mark, R.; Kavesh, W. N.; Rabkin, M. T.; Turner, B.; Bachrach, S.; and Lennox, S. "A Continuum of Care for the Inner City: Assessment of its Benefits for Boston's Elderly and High-Risk Populations." *New England Journal of Medicine* 320 (1980): 1434–40.

McKeown, T. *The Role of Medicine: Dream, Mirage, or Nemesis?* London: Nuffield Provincial Hospitals Trust, 1976.

Pollak, W. *Expanding Health Benefits for the Elderly.* Vol. 1: *Long-Term Care.* Washington, D.C.: Urban Institute, 1979.

Powers, P. *Consumer Satisfaction with Hearing Aids.* Utah State University Research Study (mimeo) 1976.

Powers, P., and Jero, A. *Sound Trap: Hearing Aid Sales in Iowa.* Iowa Student Public Interest Group, 1974.

Reid, D. W., and Ziegler, M. "A Desired Control Measure for Studying the Psychological Adjustment of the Elderly." Paper presented at the Symposium on "Goal-Specific Locus of Control Scales—A New Step in I-E Research," Annual Meeting of the American Psychological Association, Toronto, September 1, 1978 (mimeo).

Riley, M.W.; Foner, A.; Hess, B.; and Toby, M. L. "Socialization for the Middle and Later Years," in *Handbook of Socialization Theory and Research.* ed. D. A. Goslin. Chicago: Rand McNally, 1969.

Sager, A. *Improving the Provision of Non-Institutional Long-Term Care to the Elderly.* Levinson Policy Institute, Florence Heller Graduate School for Advanced Studies in Social Welfare, Waltham, Mass.: Brandeis University, 1978.

Shanas, E. "The Family as a Social Support System in Old Age." *Gerontologist* 19 (1979): 169–74.

Taylor, E. "Policy Implications of Long-Term Care for the Elderly," in *The Health Services Policy Session,* ed. M. Pollard. Washington, D.C.: Public Reference Branch of the Federal Trade Commission, 1979.

U.S. Comptroller General. *Entering a Nursing Home—Costly Implications for Medicaid and the Elderly.* PAD-80-12. Washington, D.C.: G.P.O., 1979.

Weissert, W. G.; Wan, T. T. H.; and Livieratos, B. B. *Effects and Costs of Day Care and Homemaker Services for the Chronically Ill: A Randomized Experiment.* Hyattsville, Md.: DHEW, 1979.

Williams, T. F.; Hill, J. G.; Fairbank, M. E.; and Knox, K. G. "Appropriate Placement of the Chronically Ill and Aged." *JAMA* 226 (1973): 1332–35.

4

Allocating Long-Term-Care Services
The Policy Puzzle of Who Should Be Served

Elizabeth A. Kutza

Introduction

Due to a confluence of demographic, political, and social forces, we are witnessing an increasing demand for the development of a system of long-term-care services. The phrase "long-term care" typically represents a range of services that address the health and social and personal care needs of individuals who for one reason or another have never developed or have lost some capacity for self-care. Services may be continuous or intermittent, but it is generally presumed that they will be delivered for the "long term," that is, indefinitely, to individuals who have a demonstrated need, usually measured by some index of functional incapacity. The demand for a long-term-care service system is directed primarily at the public sector, especially the federal government, whose responsibility in the provision and financing of health and social services continues to grow. Consequently, it is the nature and extent of public responsibility in this area that are now under serious debate.

While public officials eagerly engage in dialogue on the matter, they reluctantly engage in action. Their reluctance to implement a broadly based public initiative rests largely upon uncertainty of estimates as regards potential demand for such services. Who would choose to utilize a system of publicly organized and financed long-term-care services? What categories of persons would be likely beneficiaries? Answers to these and related questions about the populations-at-risk for long-term-care services remain woefully inadequate. Yet if accurate estimates of potential demand were available, we would likely find that our resources, no matter how "generous," would be unable to satisfy the demand. Thus the difficult choices remain—who can be served given limited economic and political resources (a practical consideration), and upon what basis should this selection process be based (an ethical consideration)? A major goal of this paper is to explore major determinants of these choices as well as to highlight consequences which may result from alternate choices.

**Potential Demand for and
Allocation of Long-Term-Care Services**

Because scarcity of resources is a certainty in society, rationing is requisite. In the marketplace where price is the rationing mechanism, goods and services are allocated according to consumer demand. The value of the goods or services is reflected in the price the individual consumer is willing to pay for them. Consequently at any given price, demand is estimable.

Governmentally produced or subsidized goods have no equivalently simple rationing mechanism. Public benefits are allocated by nonmarket principles. Government provides goods and services in accordance with some vision of the public good and, in the social welfare arena, in accordance with some notion of need. Sometimes, for administrative simplicity, "need" is determined presumptively.[1] Alternatively, public benefits are allocated upon "demonstrated need," either diagnostically demonstrated (blindness, mental illness) or economically demonstrated (means-tested welfare programs).

As in the market analogy, the rationing mechanism of the public program must be known in order to estimate with any accuracy potential consumer demand. Different estimates of potential demand will result from different mechanisms. If a program is developed which allocates benefits on the basis of presumed need, one estimate will prevail; if on the basis of demonstrated need, another.[2] Still a third estimate might result if projections from the pattern of demand now extant in the long-term-care arena are used. An elaboration of the limits of demand estimates, whether based on presumed need, demonstrated need, or current utilization, will highlight the policy puzzle of who should be served.

Presumed Need for Service

The likelihood of requiring long-term-care services is not shared equally among persons in society. Membership in certain categories or classes of persons significantly increases one's risk. An admittedly gross, but nonetheless reasonably good, discriminator between low-risk and high-risk categories of persons is the presence of chronic illness. Chronic illness is illness which has one or more of the following characteristics: it is permanent; it is nonreversible; it may be expected to require a long period of supervision, observation, or care. Persons with chronic illness generally experience some limit in their capacity to function independently, and such functional incapacity has significant implications for social functioning and independent living.[3]

The categories of persons who may be presumed to have some functional limitation resulting from a chronic illness or disability are several. They include those persons of advanced old age, those with physical and developmental disabilities, and those with chronic mental illness. Individuals in these groups can be identified as members of the population-at-risk for long-term-care services. They experience a level of dependency that is greater than normal. They may need supervision and aid in managing a chronic medical condition and accomplishing the routine tasks of life.

Several programs, built upon the presumed community care needs of these populations, are currently operating. They may have different names, but their service packages are identical, including provisions for health, social, and personal care. The catalog of services for the elderly are identified as long-term-care services. For the handicapped these same services are called a program of independent living, and for the mentally ill, a community support program. Each package of services is available only to a specific category of persons; each emanates from a different bureaucracy. Program development in long-term care for the elderly rests in the Health Care Financing Administration (HCFA) and the Administration on Aging (AoA). In fiscal year 1980, the two agencies shared $20 million earmarked for the development of long-term-care demonstration projects. Congress also approved $15 million in the 1980 budget to support the National Program of Independent Living of the Rehabilitation Services Administration and $6.7 million for the development of the Community Support Program of the National Institute of Mental Health through contracts with nineteen states and the District of Columbia.

The stated goals of each of these initiatives are to reduce institutionalization and encourage independent living within the community. The service package in each program includes health care, personal care, housing arrangements, housekeeping activities, counseling, and, most especially, case management. These current program commitments presume that individuals in the identified categories need a comprehensive range of community support services if they are to maintain their independence within the community. The numbers of persons within these categories or populations-at-risk, while difficult to count accurately, suggest a large potential demand for services.

Populations-at-risk

Certain classes or categories of persons may be presumed to be at risk for long-term-care services. By risk we mean that because of certain characteristics inherent in the class, persons within the class incur a greater likelihood of needing long-term-care services than persons outside the class. In the mind of many, the category of persons at greatest risk for long-term-care is the elderly. Undoubtedly, sickness is found more frequently among the old as a group than among the young as a group. Chronic age-related diseases such as arthritis and arteriosclerosis restrict mobility and memory function. But the aged are not alone in experiencing the functional limitations brought on by a chronic illness or disability. Morris observed: "Even though *the rate* of serious disablement and service need is higher for those over 65, over 75, and over 85, *the total* number who may require or could use some kind of [long-term-care] services, regardless of criteria used, seems to divide about evenly—evenly between those over and under 65 years of age."[4]

Several categories of nonaged persons could use and do receive long-term-care services of a medical, social, and personal nature, both formally through agencies and informally through family and friends. Two such nonaged categories can be readily identified—the physically and developmentally disabled, and the chronically mentally ill. Thus, gross estimates of the number of person in each of these categories will identify the populations-at-risk for long-term-care services.

Before we proceed, a word of caution is needed as regards the figures about to be cited. First, the figures presented on the aged, disabled, and mentally ill are not additive. Estimates of the disabled may include the chronically mentally ill; the chronically mentally ill may include some elderly; and the developmentally disabled include both children and adults. This double counting is a function of how these data are gathered, and the figures presented should be viewed only as approximations of reality.

Second, the presence of a chronic disease in the population-at-risk, while often associated with some functional limitation, is only one indicator among many of the need for formally organized long-term-care services. Two individuals afflicted with the same disease and experiencing the same level of functional limitation (e.g., multiple sclerosis patients who are wheelchair bound), may have available widely different adaptive mechanisms and informal supports, and thus may need very different levels of formal service.

To reiterate, these estimates of categorical populations-at-risk for long-term care have only limited value in the current policy debate. Their main purpose is to highlight that many categories of persons can be presumed to need long-term-care services.

The aged.—The elderly are seen as needing long-term-care services because age strongly relates to the presence of functional limitation. In self-report surveys of perceived disability, the proportion of people who consider themselves disabled increases with age. A Social Security Administration survey of noninstitutionalized adults aged 18 to 64 indicates that over one-half of those reporting severe disability were between the ages of 55 and 64.[5]

About 400,000 persons, or 17.3 percent of those over 65 report a functional limitation severe enough to render them unable to work or keep house.[6]

These facts, along with changing demographics, make the elderly a growing population-at-risk for long-term-care services. Presently, 11 percent of the population is over 65. Experts believe that this proportion may rise to 12.5 percent by the year 2000, and may continue to increase to as much as 16 percent by 2030.[7]

But it is not merely increases in the proportion of elderly in society that are of particular interest to long-term planners, for most people will age in reasonably good health. What is significant is the expected increase in the most vulnerable of older persons, those beyond age 75. In 1975, 8.3 million persons were over age 75 in the United States. Estimates for the year 2000 range from 11.7 million to 18.1 million persons, depending upon then-existing mortality rates.[8] These increases will push up the demand for long-term-care services, institutional and noninstitutional.

The physically and developmentally disabled.—The report of the White House Conference on the Handicapped estimates that 33 million individuals living in the United States are physically disabled owing to speech, hearing, visual, and orthopedic impairments, cerebral palsy, epilepsy, muscular distrophy, multiple sclerosis, cancer, diabetes, heart disease, mental retardation and specific learning disabilities. A more conservative estimate of the number of disabled in the country is found in the 1970 census and the 1972 Social Security Administration's Survey of the Disabled. The census counted 11.2 million persons between the ages of 16 and 64 (one in eleven persons) with functional disabilities. Of this number, approximately 1.7 million persons were homebound owing to chronic health disorders or degenerative diseases, and 2.1 million were institutionalized.[9] The SSA survey counted one in nine persons disabled (15.6 million persons between the ages of 20 and 64), including approximately 7.7 million severely disabled.[10]

Surveys of the noninstitutionalized, physically disabled adult population present the following profile. More women than men report disabilities. While blacks are only one-half as likely to be disabled as whites, they are twice as likely to be severely disabled. Almost 25 percent of all disabilities result from an accident, most frequently on the job, slightly less frequently in an automobile. Of the disabled surveyed by the Social Security Administration, most report some limitation in their ability to function independently.

Because the incidence of mental retardation cannot be ascertained with any accuracy, the profile of the developmentally disabled population is less clear. Most frequently it is estimated that 3 percent of the total population, at some time in their lives, will be considered developmentally disabled. Of the total retarded population, 89 percent is mildly retarded, 6 percent moderately retarded, and approximately 5 percent profoundly or seriously retarded.

The weakness of estimates in this area is demonstrated by the remarkable variance in the prevalence of mental retardation by chronological age. The highest prevalence occurs during school years when retardation is socially defined by routine testing. During infancy and early childhood, mild retardation usually is not apparent, and after formal schooling the mildly retarded person is capable of making a marginal adjustment to the routine demands of adulthood. The prevalence of retardation during adulthood is further reduced by the relatively high preadult mortality rate among the more severely and profoundly retarded.[11] Because of this variability, Tarjan and his associates argue that only 1 percent of the total population should be considered mentally retarded for purposes of programming.[12] Upon this estimate, about 210,000 moderately to severely retarded persons could be presumed to need ongoing supportive services.

It is not known whether physical and developmental disabilities among adults are on the rise in American society, but it is apparent that the number of persons who qualify for public benefits on the basis of disability is increasing. The number of workers who qualify for disability insurance benefits, for example, has doubled in seven years. During fiscal 1977 alone, more than 1.2 million workers filed disability claims. While 60 percent of the claims were denied, 185,750 denied disability cases were appealed to administrative law judges, and another 18,000 are pending in the federal courts.[13] While many provisions in the program itself have contributed to this increase, the experiences of privately financed disability plans and of government programs in other countries generally have paralleled those of the Social Security program. Hence, one conclusion might be that the public acceptance of the government's role in compensating for the functional limitations brought about by disability is growing.

Since most of the data thus far presented on the disabled were drawn from surveys of adults, it is important to draw out another subset of the disabled population, children with chronic diseases. With improved treatment of infectious diseases and increased ability to sustain life without restoring health, there is a growing number of children who suffer from severe and chronic illness. Medical management of such conditions is limited. A physician may be able to control the rate of progression or the frequency and severity of complications of the disease, but successful management of the more destructive secondary effects of chronic illness in children requires a complete package of supportive, counseling, coordinative, and educational services.

Estimates of the prevalence of chronic illness among children vary. A rough working estimate of the most prevalent conditions handicapping children and their probable incidence in 1980 is as follows: about 3 million children suffer from congenital heart disease, and another 2.6 million from orthopedic handicaps; 500,000 children have epilepsy, and an equal number cerebral palsy, and over 100,000 suffer from childhood diabetes.[14]

While the availability of preventive measures (e.g., family planning, avoidance of x-rays during pregnancy, nutrition programs for low-income mothers, prenatal care for high-risk mothers) may result eventually in a decrease in the number of handicapped children, progress is slow. The National Foundation of the March of Dimes estimates that in 1979 close to 2 million children under the age of 20 were living with the results of a birth defect, and over 100,000 infants were newly affected.[15] Soon, however, genetic counseling may sharply reduce the number of children born with hereditary birth defects. Mass screening procedures are being developed that identify such defects *in utero,* thus allowing parents to terminate the pregnancy. (The ethical dilemmas associated with advanced technology in this area remain to be resolved.)

But genetic abnormality is not the only source of chronic illness in children. Another is low birth weight. Five and a half pounds is generally considered the dividing line between normal and low birth weight. Some 7 percent (230,000 annually) of American newborns weigh 5½ pounds or less. These dangerously small infants often have severe problems with breathing, heart action, and regulation of temperature and blood sugar. Unless these difficulties are controlled, they may cause brain damage or death. Structural defects occur in about 6 percent of babies weighing more than 5½ pounds; in 9 percent of those between 4 lb. 7 oz. and 5 lb. 8 oz; and in more than 30 percent of those weighing 4 lb. 6 oz. or less. Thus, low birth weight is the most common birth defect of all and is the major cause of disability in childhood.[16] And the incidence of low-birth-weight newborns is especially high among teenaged mothers.

Each year nearly a quarter of a million American girls have babies before their eighteeenth birthday, and the babies of these young mothers are more likely to develop the neurological disabilities and mental retardation associated with low birth weight. One study found the incidence of retardation in children born to mothers under age 17 to be nearly five times the proportion in the general population.[17] Poor nutrition and poor prenatal care are the main reasons these infants either are born prematurely or sustain impaired fetal growth. Thus, the recent progress in combating the chronic diseases of childhood caused by genetic abnormality may be in jeopardy because of the increasing numbers of high-risk infants born to teenaged women.

The mentally ill.—As a result of the mandates of the Community Mental Health Center Construction Act of 1963, thousands of mentally ill persons were transferred from institutional settings back to their own communities to receive care. Before this law was enacted, 75 percent of all the people who received care were residents of the institutions in which they received that care. Now, according to the President's Commission on Mental Health, three of every four persons receiving formal mental health care are outpatients in public and private settings.[18]

While the community mental health ideology was based on beliefs that community care would save money, that continuity of care would be enhanced, that former patients would be rehabilitated, and that the mentally ill would be integrated into society, these hopes have not been fulfilled. Klerman has referred to deinstitutionalized patients as "better but not well," and he notes their need for some degree of social support, e.g., welfare or disability payments, special residential placements, and social supervision, usually in day care programs.[19] The number of severely chronically mentally disabled adults who, while not in need of 24-hour nursing care, do need supportive services of an indefinite duration has been estimated at 1.5 million nationwide.[20]

Three categories of persons—the very old, the disabled, and the mentally ill—have been identified here as potential candidates for the receipt of long-term-care services. While estimates of the numbers of persons in each group are not additive and the categories overlap, there is no doubt that serving all who presumably could use long-term-care services requires a vast program, so vast that it is likely to be economically and politically unfeasible. If that is the case, then estimates drawn from populations-at-risk for long-term-care services are of little help in deciding who is to be served.

Demonstrated Need for Long-Term-Care Services

If presumed need is an unsatisfactory basis upon which to allocate long-term-care services, what other criterion can be used? One possibility is "demonstrated need." Under this allocative principle, only persons who can demonstrate a need for the service, as reflected in some index of incapacity, would be counted within the population to be served. Generating estimates of the number of such persons and their demand for services is difficult, however, because of measurement problems.

Measuring need.—The concept of need remains a puzzling one for program planners. Economists, for example, regard need as a normative reflection of individual values and wishes. Because need is normative it defies attempts at standardized measurement. An illustration will highlight the problem.

Civil libertarians and classical economists argue that the individual is the best judge of his/her own need (i.e., preference) for service. Excluding those cases in which there is a highly specialized question of medical management, as well as those cases in which the individual in question may be of limited mental capacity, the typical consumer seems capable of judging his/her own needs. In the long-term-care area, where service needs address living arrangements, tasks of daily living, and personal care, the argument seems supportable. Yet self-report surveys of needs are notoriously poor guides for developing new public services.[21] For what a person "objectively" needs and will use may be modified by his personality (dependent v. independent), his motivation, and his ingenuity at simplifying his life into a more manageable arrangement. Thus personal standards of needs and wants are too variable to be of much use to program planners.

Alternative to this self-report approach, or more usually adjunctive to it, estimates of need have come from outside observers who assess level of functioning on a case-by-case basis. The level of functional incapacity is then used as a proxy for the need for long-term-care services.

Over the years, large numbers of functional assessment tools have been developed. By functional assessment is meant "any systematic attempt to measure objectively the level at which the person is functioning, in any of a variety of areas such as physical health, quality of self maintenance, quality of role activity, intellectual status, social activity, attitude toward the world and toward self, and emotional status."[22] Indexes of functional limitations generally operationalize and measure an individual's capacity for self care by assessing his ability to perform activities of daily living (bathing, dressing, eating, walking) and instrumental activities of daily living (using the telephone, shopping, doing laundry).

The major shortcoming of functional assessment tools is that the level of functioning they measure is not readily translated into need for service. For example, a person may score poorly on mobility. A response to that problem can take various forms—a wheelchair, a walker, a cane, better shoes, podiatry services. Kleh notes the essential lack in the long-term-care field of an appropriate scheme for classifying patients in terms of service needs.[23] Because of this lack, the judgment of service need rests with the professional service workers, each of whom may apply different standards. In studies comparing the status of institutionalized and noninstitutionalized elderly, for example, differential levels of functional ability have been found to be poor predictors of placement. In 1975, a long-term-care study done in Illinois estimated that about 33 percent of the clients receiving community care (not necessarily formal) had limitations that met or exceeded those of elderly in long-term-care institutions.[24]

Yet the traditional importance to program planners of estimating need for service is clear. Answers to questions such as who needs service (by age, sex, race, location), what type of service they need, how much or how often they need service, are relevant to decisions about program eligibility, service delivery mechanisms, and financing. Without such data, service development and manpower projections are risky. To date, however, we know very little about the level of demonstrated need for long-term-care services in American society, and we know even less about how that need may distribute itself throughout the society.

Current Demand for Long-Term-Care Services

The need of individuals for supportive services in the management of chronic illness whether assessed on the basis of demonstrated functional limitation or on the basis of categorical presumption is only suggestive of the potential demand for formally organized services. The foregoing data merely hint at the kinds and numbers of persons who *might* use such services, not who should or would. But we do know something about the current demand for already existing services and, by implication, these data may tell us who is most in need of, i.e., most values, these services.

As has already been noted, the level of demand for services of any kind in our market economy is set by a complex mixture of individual preferences and the price of the service. While studies are still needed which experimentally vary price so as better to understand the relationship between demand and cost of long-term-care services, some studies have been done which aim at understanding current utilization of existing services, that is, how much of the service is actually used. Andersen and Newman's work on utilization of medical care, for example, identifies three interrelated factors which explain differential use of service: predisposing factors, such as family attitudes, social structure, and health beliefs; enabling factors, such as family and community resources; "need," including both the illness and the individual's perception of it.[25] In the long-term-care area, research is just beginning to untangle these correlates of utilization, and to identify the most important ones.

Utilization figures for community-based support services are poor indicators of demand because of the limited supply of such services now available. Only 10 percent of all public financing for long-term-care services goes to support noninstitutional arrangements. Thus the important policy question is what would be the demand for services *if* a fully matured system of community supports were made available. As Pollak points out, "if broad coverage is provided, . . . community care will flow to two distinct groups. First, there are those who would then live in the community but who now reside in institutions, either because needed community care services are not financed and available or because in the absence of such services, these persons' conditions deteriorate to the point at which institutionalization is dictated. Second there are those who already live in the community. Most of the care they now receive is provided informally by spouse, other relatives, or friends. . . . [Additionally are other] impaired persons in the community [who] need but do not now receive any care, either from programs or from kin."[26]

These latter groups of potential beneficiaries may be quite large, although reliable estimates of how many people who are not now receiving services would take advantage of public long-term-care services should they become more widespread are unavailable. Powers and Bultana, studying the correspondence between anticipated and actual uses of public services by the aged, report that earlier statements of personal need and willingness to use public programs are not a good indicator of later behavior. They asked a group of older persons to list those service programs they thought should be provided in their communities, and those they would personally use. Eleven years later, the living respondents were reinterviewed. They were asked how available these resources had become in their community, and how much they used them. No more than nine percent of the 600 persons in sample were actually using the services in 1971 that they said they needed and would use in 1960.[27] Thus even when researchers inquire about service use from potential populations-at-risk, the findings bring them no closer to estimates of potential utilization.

While little is known about the ultimate utilization of an extensive community care system, data are available on whether a disabled person receives care in the community or within an institution. In these studies "need," or health status, has been found to be a poor predictor of placement. Most attention has been focused on Andersen and Newman's "enabling factors," community and family supports.

Obviously, if few formal resources exist within a community, utilization will be low. Additionally, community attitudes about how the elderly are to be served and by whom affect the development of community resources. Pollak, for example, observes intriguing differences in interstate variability of nursing home utilization. After adjusting for the age structure of the elderly population in each state, he developed an index to measure the propensity of a state to use nursing homes. Real differences emerged in the way the care problems of the elderly were handled among states. Unfortunately the data do not explain the differences found. Thus it is unknown, for example, "whether low utilization rates in a state were due to unusual propensities of families to care for their old, to high availability of home care, to the substitution of boarding home care for nursing home care or to some other factor."[28] So while it is fairly certain that community attitudes and resources affect the supply and demand of long-term-care services, there remain interesting questions for future research.

The existence of social supports is another variable which influences the utilization of formal long-term-care services. Increasingly, studies identify a community network as key in explaining differences in utilization of long-term-care services. This network may involve neighbors, family, or friends who regularly give and receive objects, services, social and emotional supports.[29] Whether the individual is a retarded child or a frail older person, the willingness of these informal support networks to provide ongoing care is critical to keeping the person out of the formal service delivery system.

As regards health-related tasks, including emergency assistance, and the more long-range personal care commitment of daily bathing, giving medicine, and transportation to the doctor, the role of the family is clear.[30] For the functionally limited adult, the main source of support is the spouse. The importance of the spouse is reflected in nursing home resident data that show three times as high a proportion of persons who have never been married and twice as high a proportion of widowed persons. Children, both within and outside of the household, are the next sources of help. Childless and low-fertility women have a 15 percent higher chance of institutionalization before age 75 than do women who bore three or more children.[31]

Going beyond the family, Cantor and Johnson explored the extent and relative roles of friends and neighbors in the provision of personalized, individualized home care. Sampling from a universe of all persons 60 and older living in New York's inner city ($n = 1,552$), they found only 15 percent of their sample (234 persons) without at least one "functional kin."[32] This subgroup was called "familyless." Of those classified as "familyless," 74 percent had functional neighbors or friends. (A functional friend was seen at least monthly, and was in phone contact at least weekly; a functional neighbor was known well by the respondent, and interacted with the respondent in one or more instrumental or affective ways). Thus, only 4 percent of the total sample of New York City's elderly were without viable supports. While these elderly—those without "functional kin"—showed no greater frailty, they were more likely to be found living alone; there was a higher proportion of men to women; and they were poorer than others in the sample. They also suffered from lower morale and sense of well-being.[33]

Hence a critical variable that explains why individuals of similar age, with similar levels of income and functional ability are residing in different settings is living arrangement, primarily in the form of living with spouse and/or children, or living in a community with available functional relatives, neighbors, or friends.

But informal caretaking arrangements may be fragile, as evidenced by a study done in New England. The cases of almost 300 patients from four rehabilitation facilities were followed upon discharge. "For patients in the study population who went into institutions rather than into their own homes" the study notes, "it was found that following a previous episode of hospitalization, family members had provided care at home for 70 percent of the patients. After this second hospitalization, families of only 38 percent of the patients were willing to give such care. On the other hand, for those who were hospitalized for the first time, the proportion of relatives who had given care prior to hospitalization was 44 percent, and 63 percent of families indicated willingness to provide care on the patients' discharge."[34] The researchers conclude that formal long-term-care provisions may be necessary to underpin and sustain a high level of family care. In the absence of a formal system, family capacity is rapidly eroded, leading to a situation in which institutional care is completely substituted for family care.

In summary the data on utilization help us understand why those who use formally provided services opt for institutional or noninstitutional arrangements. These decisions are influenced by supply factors within different communities; individual, community, and professional attitudes about the most appropriate modes of caring for disabled individuals; and willingness of informal support networks to assume the task of caring. While interesting, these modifiers of utilization rates provide little basis upon which to estimate potential demand for long-term-care services. Whatever the baseline demand, however, it is likely to increase as certain trends which promote utilization are continuing.

Influences on Future Demand

Several sociological and demographic changes in American society are accelerating whatever demand now exists for formally provided long-term-care services. Some of these changes, especially the rising proportion of the very old and the alteration of family structures and roles, will increase demand for all types of long-term-care services. Other changes, such as the growing societal preference for deinstitutionalization and the increasing militancy of disabled groups, specifically will increase demand for community-based and home-based services. All of these changes have begun, and their impact can be explored.

As an increasing proportion of Americans live into advanced old age, the demand for long-term-care services will grow. The significant effect on social policy of having more persons of advanced age in the society is clear. People over 75 are three times more likely to need personal care assistance than those between the ages of 65 and 74, and nursing home utilization increases with age. Pollak has estimated that 9.1 percent of the elderly between 80 and 84 and 16.6 percent of the elderly over 85 are residents of nursing homes. For the age categories 65 to 69 and 70 to 74 the comparable estimates are one and two percent, respectively.[35]

Increased demand for organized long-term-care services will also grow out of changes in family structure and roles. As earlier noted, community studies repeatedly document the essential role of the family in meeting the long-term-care needs of disabled individuals. In the case of disabled children, the parent, especially the mother, is the primary caretaker. For the adult invalid, the spouse is the main source of help, followed by children (within and outside the household), siblings, other kind, and friends. But in the future, this network of caretakers may be less available for several reasons.

First, as more women are employed outside the home, fewer will be available for full-time caretaking activities. Forty million women (49 percent of all women over 16 years of age) are now in the labor force. While middle-aged women were largely responsible for increases in labor force participation between 1950 and 1965, the largest gains have now shifted to women under age 35. In fact, the Labor Department labels "phenomenal" the increase that has been occurring among women 25 to 34 years of age. Their labor force participation rates advanced by 12 percentage points between 1970 and 1976, a remarkable increase since the majority of women in this age group are married, live with their husbands, and have children at home, factors which traditionally have tended to keep women out of the labor force.[36]

Most of these women work because of economic necessity. On average, wives' earnings account for 26 percent of the total family income, and as much as 39 percent in families where wives worked year round, full time. Thus if wives discontinued working so as to care for a disabled child or older person, family well-being would suffer. Middle-aged wives especially, accustomed to the social stimulation and economic gains of outside employment, only reluctantly might forego these things to care for an aging parent or in-law.

Not only changing family roles, but also changing family structures are affecting caretaking presumptions. Four-generation families are no longer unusual. Within such families, the very old invalid has children who themselves are struggling with the chronic debilitations of old age. Alternatively, an old person may outlive his/her children, siblings, and friends and may be left with few alternatives to formal long-term-care services. Glick notes that persons in the midst of old age today are about 75 years of age. "When they were born," he says, "the average family had five children, the next generation had an average of three children; and the current generation, now in the midst of childbearing, is likely to have an average of two children."[37]

One conclusion drawn from these data is that the potential amount of mutual responsibility and natural support between successive generations is significantly altering. Future elderly may have fewer family supports available than do today's elderly, and therefore may demand the development of more formal organized services, institutional and noninstitutional.

Concurrent with these social and demographic changes is an attitudinal shift in society. There is a growing belief among professionals and the public-at-large that segregated, institutional placement for the treatment of infirmity, mental illness, and mental retardation is undesirable. Until very recently, a different attitude prevailed. It was assumed that dependent persons in need of special care should be segregated from the larger society. Removal of such persons from a milieu in which they could not compete, and placement in a sheltered, protective environment, were deemed humane. Thus we had asylums for orphans and the mentally ill, homes for the aged and infirm, and "schools" for the retarded. Gradually such placement has come under scrutiny. The value of reintegration in the community is being affirmed. Today this preference for deinstitutionalization and community-based service systems is further supported by court orders which mandate treatment in the least restrictive environment.

Most litigation has affected treatment of the mentally ill and developmentally disabled. The segregation of the mentally retarded in large isolated institutions, for example, has been subject to attack under the equal protection clause of the fourteenth amendment. Institutionalization infringes upon many rights which the Supreme Court has recognized as "fundamental," including the right to travel freely, the right to privacy, and, in some cases, the right to marry and to have children. Thus the courts have contributed to decisions affirming the right to treatment per se, and the right to treatment in the least restrictive environment.

In addition to the courts, lawmakers have indicated a preference for "deinstitutionalization." Laws affecting psychiatric treatment, education, and living arrangements have been enacted which encourage community integration.[38] Each of these laws places special demands on the Department of Health and Human Services to develop new community services. As regards services for the aged, recent nursing home scandals also push for the development of community "alternatives to institutionalization."

Accompanying this attitude shift regarding the preferred way to treat dependent groups is the new militancy of persons in these groups themselves. The original impetus to treat the infirm and mentally afflicted within the community came from professionals who witnessed the debilitating effects of segregation—low morale, excessive dependency, social isolation, and, often, mistreatment. Now, however, clients themselves are demanding such services. The aged and disabled are the newest groups to follow the lead of blacks, welfare mothers, and women, who, in pursuit of civil rights, have applied political and judicial pressure so as to increase their access to facilities, services, and opportunities. Increasingly the demands of these groups focus upon independence-enhancing, community-based social services.

These trends then—an increase in the very old, a changing family structure, a new attitude toward treatment, and a new insistence regarding the right to services—are likely to increase the demand for social provisions of a long-term-care nature. While not certain, this outcome is probable.

Conclusions

We have now reviewed what is and is not known about the need of, and potential demand for, long-term-care services in the United States. Throughout the review, the necessary and sufficient conditions of risk for the receipt of long-term-care services were noted, and the factors related to service demand and utilization were explored. On the basis of these data, certain observations can be made and conclusions drawn:

1. There remain serious questions about who needs care. Disability or functional limitation appears to be a necessary but not sufficient condition of risk for long-term care. Not all persons within high-risk categories (the very old, the disabled, the chronically mentally ill) are dependent upon others for care, and those who are dependent have needs that vary in intensity, duration, and scope. Thus whether a person "needs" long-term-care services seems more related to whether he wants them, feels he needs them, or has been advised by others that he needs them, than to some indisputable measure of need.

2. The potential demand for publicly supported long-term-care services is vast and unlikely to be fully met. Thus the rationing of benefits remains a political decision. Who should be served is a value-laden question whose resolution rests in the political arena.

3. Utilization of formally organized long-term-care services is influenced by individual preferences and informal community supports. If the prevailing attitude is that publicly provided long-term-care services are a right, an entitlement, demand will be high. Alternatively, if the prevailing attitude is that the appropriate locus of responsibility for care

rests within the family, demand will be low. These difficult-to-measure modifiers continue to make estimates of potential demand uncertain at best.

4. Whatever the current level of demand and utilization is, it will rise as a result of certain inevitable demographic and social trends. These trends include the changing age structure of society, the changing composition of the family, the changing role of women, and the changing societal outlook on community care for dependent groups.

Economic and Ethical Implication in the Allocation of Long-Term-Care Services

Estimates of need and demand for long-term-care services have direct implications for program planning. If accurate estimates are impossible, and even conservative guesses alarmingly high, program design must incorporate rationing devices that are built upon economic principles of equity and efficiency, and are rooted in ethical and legal mandates.

A series of questions will highlight the range of economic and ethical decisions that face program planners. Each question raises an issue as regards the allocation and rationing of services; each question emanates from the data reviewed in the first half of this essay. The questions posed are illustrative, not exhaustive.

Questions Having Economic Implications

1. What level of societal resources will be allocated for the purpose of long-term care?

The level of resources allocated to any social welfare area reflects an underlying view of the role of the state vis-a-vis its dependent populations. Of all Western industrialized nations, the United States has accepted most slowly and cautiously its public responsibility for dependency. Until recently, blame for social problems was attributed to the individual rather than societal circumstances. Even today this view is evident in the belief that the disadvantaged and victimized—whether by poverty, rape, unemployment, infirmity, or dependent old age—have primarily themselves to blame. The attitude has made America a "reluctant welfare state," in the words of Wilensky and Lebeaux, reluctant to provide generous and universal social services.[39]

Efforts to develop a large-scale, public program of long-term care are influenced by this reluctance. To date, for example, there is no widespread agreement as regards the role of government in the provision and financing of health care. As a result, America has no system of national health insurance. In the absence of a fundamental acceptance of the role of government in the funding of specialized health care services, there is little chance that the nonspecialized, personal care services needed by chronically ill populations will be supported.

Our concern is economic as well as philosophic; medical and personal care services are costly and difficult to deliver efficiently. As we enter a period of restrained economic growth, the philosophic attitude will be reinforced by economic realities. Thus the political decision of how many economic resources the society is willing to allocate to this one among competing alternatives becomes crucial.

2. Is it more efficient to organize long-term-care services generically or categorically, that is, by populations-at-risk?

Categorical populations-at-risk for long-term-care services all suffer from chronic illness affecting the individual's functional independence. Thus many service needs among chronically ill populations are common. They all have medical needs, for example, usually of a medical management or rehabilitative nature. On occasion the chronically ill person may suffer from an acute medical incident, or require the services of the specialist (pediatrician, geriatrician, or psychiatrist), but the common medical management needs (nursing, medication) are substantively noncategorical.

In addition to medical services, individuals in each of these groups need a range of social/psychological services. Regardless of the cause of the functional limitation—birth defect, childhood disease, work-related accident, or the progressive deterioration of the normal aging process—acceptance of limitation requires external support. Enforced and involuntary dependency alters social relations and feelings of self-worth. The individual and his/her family are confronted with service provider bureaucracies that are confusing, complex, and intimidating. The need of all long-term-care populations-at-risk for advice, encouragement, and counseling is shared, and can be provided through a generic service agency.

Services of a personal care nature also compensate for an individual's limitation of functioning. A very old or severely disabled person may need help dressing and bathing, while a less-disabled person may require aid in shopping, housecleaning, and taking a walk. At present most of these services are provided by family, neighbors, and friends, but irrespective of who provides them, they constitute a common service need for functionally limited individuals.

Recognition of the common service needs of the chronically ill and disabled is not a denial of the specialized needs of persons within certain categories. The physically disabled, for example, may require specially equipped transportation facilities that the mentally impaired do not. Protective services, in the form of guardianship, conservatorship, or enforced treatment, are appropriate for only a small subset of the long-term-care population, those whose physical or mental impairments preclude effective management of their estates, or care for themselves. Specialized education services are more directly responsive to the needs of the chronically ill or disabled child than adult, while vocational training is more relevant to the needs of the adult than the very old.

These specialized needs notwithstanding, most long-term-care service requirements of a medical, social, and personal care nature are common among chronically ill populations. Thus a universal, that is, consolidated noncategorical long-term-care service system might be efficient and should be discussed. A review of the advantages and disadvantages of one system over another is enlightening but not conclusive. On the one hand, a universal system embodies the merits of rational service delivery. It avoids duplication, fills gaps, and uses scarce resources efficiently. An individual client in such a system will not be segmented or fall through a categorical crack. Equity is better served because persons of equal need are rendered equal service.

Counterweighing these advantages are the serious bureaucratic and political problems that a reorganization of the current categorical service system would face. Existing administrative agencies only reluctantly would relinquish authority over programs and services now in their domain. Special interest groups, no longer able to target their activities to constituent agencies, would resent becoming weakened advocates. Additionally, the consolidation of a long-term-care budget in one agency highlights the politically explosive issue of cost. A several-billion-dollar budget draws less scrutiny divided among three or four agencies (even if they are providing identical services) than it does resting in one place. Thus opportunities for growth constrict with consolidation . Finally, consolidation creates a large new bureaucratic structure abounding with management problems. In sum development of a noncategorical long-term-care system in lieu of a narrowly categorical one has trade-offs. Futher public debate of the question is needed, debate which weighs the economic efficiency benefits against the political and bureaucratic costs.

3. What part should income and asset testing play in the rationing of scarce, publicly provided long-term-care services?

The treatment of income and assets in allocating public services is a complex and contentious issue among social policy planners. Income testing in public programs is meant to ensure that only those who cannot afford to purchase needed goods and services in the open market will benefit from public subsidy. Advocates for income testing argue that target efficiency in increased in such programs, a desirable outcome that maximizes scarce resources. Unfortunately, this desirable outcome is compromised by the legacies that attend income-tested programs, legacies of charity and the notorious Poor Laws. As Marmor notes, these legacies include "a combination of unappealing associations connected with intrusive investigation of needs, invasion of privacy, and loss of citizenship rights."[40] Stigma also accompanies such programs because income testing draws sharp distinctions between beneficiaries and non-beneficiaries. At a recent conference that addressed the merits of income-tested vs. universal programs, Garfinkel concludes: "Income-tested programs will always be vulnerable to definitions that are stig-matizing to beneficiaries and therefore, involve a cost to them which reduces the value of the benefit they are receiving."[41]

But income and asset criteria may be suitable for allocating long-term-care services. Data have long demonstrated that the functionally disabled are overrepresented among the very poor. Almost 40 percent of all the functionally disabled, and close to 70 percent of all those functionally disabled who are residing in institutions, had incomes of less than $3,000 in 1975.[42] Several factors interact to explain this phenomenon, mainly education level, age, and sex.

Compounding the problem of low income is the high cost associated with the management of a chronic illness. Even families of modest means suffer economic hardship as they provide for the special service needs of a disabled member. For these reasons, income and asset tests have been regarded as reasonable eligibility criteria for the receipt of long-term-care services.

Advocates for the elderly and disabled, increasingly vocal about their rights to services, object to income-tested programs, and may apply political pressure to resist such eligibility criteria. Yet, income and asset testing has long been considered a sensible rationing mechanism for public social benefits, and needs serious consideration in the long-term-care debate.

4. To what extent should the presence of informal supports (family, friends) affect the level of public benefits allocated to a person in need of long-term-care?

As pressure for publicly funded, in-home services increases, questions arise about the interplay between organized services and the care pro-vided by informal supports. Findings of a recent study done by the Community Services Society of New York lead Frankfather, et al., to note: "If strong anti-nursing home sentiment explains a substantial opposition of family commitment, then the emergence of an attractive alternative would have a strong impact on the family."[43] Thus Brody argues, "If retention of the disabled in the community is a public goal ... support of the family caring unit should become a critical consideration that governs policy-making in the field of long term care."[44]

Families that care for a chronically ill family member at home are under great stress. For spouses of disabled persons, role overload becomes a problem. Fengler and Goodrich summarize the situation faced by many: "A low income obviously reduces access to means that may make living with a handicapped person more bearable. It also enhances the likelihood that a wife must work. . . . For the employed wives, putting in a full day of work and then coming home to a husband [child or parent] who needs a great deal of care is extremely tiring."[45]

A recent study of all geriatric admissions to two London hospitals found that 12 percent were patients whose relatives or friends could no longer cope with them at home. In 80 percent of the cases the dependent's behavior patterns were identified as the main source of stress (e.g., sleep disturbances). In 12 percent of the cases it was the supporter's own limitations (e.g., anxiety and depression); and in the remaining 8 percent, environmental and social conditions were identified as the principal problem most poorly tolerated (e.g., restricted social life).[46]

Since family caretaking is an important source of service for the functionally impaired, new policies should aim to support, not supplant, family effort. Litwak suggests that the family and formal service providers share functions.[47] The family is good at providing nonspecialized, non-routine tasks, while formal service providers are better at meeting the specialized, routine needs of long-term-care patients. Thus, maximization of available resources requires a partnership.

Moroney, in his influential work on *The Family and the State* argues that many social policies are built upon explicit assumptions about the role of the family toward its dependent members. "Families," he says, "who are willing to provide care will be expected to carry the total burden until they no longer can." Organized services are seen as residual, taking over when the family fails. As a result, Moroney notes, social services that attempt to support the family receive lower priority than those that replace the family.[48] In planning long-term-care services, then, perhaps the client of service should be the family, not merely the disabled individual.

Questions Having Ethical and Legal Implications

1. Who should receive public long term care benefits?

If resources are scarce and potential demand great, who should be served? Lipman in a discussion of the ethics of resource allocation observes: "When we deal with competing values at this level, we are not discussing the difference between what is right and what is wrong, but between what is right and what is more right. For example, both the aged and the young need and deserve support; if higher allocations to one result in a lower share to another group—a premise we have established as being implicit when dealing with scarce resources—then which group gets the larger share, or should the shares be equal?"[49]

Choosing to serve one group, thereby excluding another, is routine in social welfare programming. Historically, eligibility for service has been based upon attributed need (e.g., age), severity of need, and low income. Any of these criteria can be used to allocate long-term-care services, but each has limitations.

Let us consider the ethical issues of using age to allocate public benefits. Clearly age, as such, is not a morally relevant characteristic. Diggs notes: "It is not clear that there are any really significant moral requirements owed to older people simply because they are old."[50] Yet age as a basis upon which to allocate long-term-care services has merit. It is straightforward to determine. The medical component of a long-term-care package can be funded through the existing Medicare program. The need for personal care services and the risk of institutionalization increase with age. Age seventy-five seems to be the turning point at which the debilitation caused by the aging process is directly reflected in increased service utilization. By the evidence, eligibility for long-term-care services, if set at age seventy or seventy-five, would effectively ration services. And, until very recently, no legal restrictions were placed upon using age as a criterion for allocating public benefits. But the enactment of the Age Discrimination Act (89 Stat. 713) may change this in the future.

Although enacted in 1975, the Age Discrimination Act is not yet fully implemented. The final regulations were not published until June 1979. As a result, its impact is not clear. While the intent of the statute would seem to prohibit discrimination on the basis of age in programs receiving federal assistance, exempted from coverage are those age distinctions contained in a program or activity "established under the authority of any law" (Sec. 90.1). Thus Title XVIII of the Social Security Act (Medicare), which contains a statutory age distinction, is exempt.

While formerly enacted statutes are not affected, the Age Discrimination Act does affect new laws. At the very least, the Act forces Congress to examine closely each new statute that attempts to use an age criterion to restrict program benefit receipt. If the use of age cannot be defended, it must be rejected. In the context of the long-term-care debate, programs that restrict service to an over-65 population are challengeable by non-aged disabled groups. The Age Discrimination Act gives such challenges increased force. Thus, while the Act does not prohibit use of age in deciding who should be served, it highlights the use of age as a matter for debate on a program by program basis.

Severity of need is another criterion upon which services are restricted. Long-term-care services, for example, can be restricted to those whose functional limitation is severe, and who have no alternative informal supports. This strategy embodies an ethical posture of the government as provider of last resort. It supports the belief that the individual and his family have an obligation to remain independently functioning, without public provision, until no other option exists. But if no other option exists, from a moral point of view such persons make a special call on our benevolence. And in the name of justice, the society chooses to respond.

In sum, choices about who to serve, and how to restrict eligibility for program benefits, are complex. They are full of ethical and legal trade-offs. While difficult, they are unavoidable.

2. How long should be the "long term"?

As medical advances extend the life of children born with birth defects, patients with terminal illness, and severely incapacitated aged, the "end stage" of long-term-care services becomes an issue. Maintenance services to those whose condition has stabilized may go on indefinitely, although, if rehabilitative, at a declining rate. Among several hundred rehabilitation hospital discharges who were given a home-care-service regime, for example, the demand for home care actually decreased after six months. The education for self-maintenance that occurred obviously allowed the disabled person to take better care of himself.[51]

But for those who have no hope of recovery or rehabilitation, for those who require costly and continuous care, more serious questions of resource allocation arise.

Should life be sustained at any cost? Children today, born with spina bifida (an opening in the spine) or hydrocephalus (water on the brain), are kept alive in high-technology, neonatal nurseries. These children cannot survive without the sophisticated care provided there. Yet when they do survive, their needs for care remain high. In 1979, over 6,000 such youngsters were newly affected, and about 53,000 children under age twenty suffered from these conditions. The costs of keeping such children alive in the early months of life, and providing them with services if they survive, are enormous. (The daily charge for intensive care in the neonatal clinic of Wyler's Children's Hospital in Chicago, for example, is about $500.00). How many resources should be expended on these youngsters who may never reach adulthood? At the other end of the age spectrum are the very old, whose progressive deterioration is irreversible. What is our view about keeping the very old alive?

While as a society we seem to stand firmly against such "primitive" practices as killing deformed infants or sending old people off to die on an ice floe, movements that support abortion of the fetus with defects, and euthanasia for the very old, are beginning. California recently passed the country's first right-to-die bill for terminally ill patients, indicating, perhaps, the public's growing acceptance of passive euthanasia. The extension of life, especially if accomplished through the expenditure of public funds, is a basic yet contentious issue facing long-term-care planners.

3. How can a long-term-care service system be developed that respects the legal and personal rights of individuals?

Since long-term-care services under a national program would affect the daily lives of many functionally impaired persons, they should be delivered in a humane and independence-enhancing manner. For example, persons in need of such services should be allowed to remain in their homes and communities, not sent to isolating institutions. Increasingly, the prevailing view is that institutional commitment should be limited to those for whom community care would be unfeasible, that is, too difficult to deliver and too costly. More important than society's growing preference for this view and its ethical appeal are recent legal decisions regarding right to treatment.

Legal doctrine underlying the right to treatment or habilitation rests upon several different, but related, legal theories. Analytically, the doctrine has passed through several stages. First, conditions in institutions were found to be so dehumanizing as to violate the rights to be free from cruel and unusual punishment (the right to freedom from harm). Then, the definition of "harm" was expanded so that a right to a constitutional minimum of services was found; finally, constitutional principles dictate that these services be provided in the least restrictive setting appropriate to the individual.[52]

Under the Constitution, the courts have held a right to treatment under the due process clause of the fourteenth amendment,[53] the eighth-amendment prohibition of cruel and unusual punishment,[54] and the equal protection clause.[55] These cases affirm the right of mentally retarded and mentally ill persons to receive adequate and appropriate services while resident in state institutions. Yet some argue that these landmark cases, which focus primarily upon conditions inside the institutions, must now be expanded to challenge the practice of institutionalization itself.

Persons needing treatment have a legal right to receive such treatment in the least restrictive environment. This right is built upon the constitutional proscription against the government's taking away more of an individual's freedom than is necessary to achieve a legitimate government goal. The current state of the law as regards least restrictive alternatives is illustrated by two recent right-to-habilitation suits. *Horacek* v. *Exon* and *Halderman* v. *Pennhurst State School and Hospital.*[56]

The complaint in *Horacek,* filed by residents of the state institution, alleged that the state of Nebraska was operating a dual system of services in violation of the fourteenth amendment. Some of the state's mentally retarded were served in a system of community services, while others were confined to Beatrice State School, the state institution for the mentally retarded. The plaintiffs contended that the system of community services was a more appropriate and less restrictive means of serving Nebraska's mentally retarded, and that continued use of Beatrice State School could not be justified.

Pennhurst involved a massive right-to-habilitation suit brought against Pennhurst State School in Pennsylvania. The court issued a sweeping order imposing strict constitutional mandates upon state officials when interfering with the liberty of the mentally retarded. In a key ruling, this court held that the state had "a constitutional duty to explore and provide the least stringent practicable alternatives to confinement of retarded individuals at Pennhurst." These cases recognize the obligation of the state to create alternative community placements for treatment and habilitation.

Most of these cases involve the rights of persons involuntarily committed for treatment. which of these constitutional guarantees apply to residents of institutions who are there voluntarily? Those courts that have addressed the issue have ruled that "voluntary" commitments are often not voluntary at all, owing to the closed nature of the institution (locked doors), the inability of many residents to consent to institutionalization or effectively to request release, the invalidity of third-party consent (parent or guardian), and the lack of community services as alternatives to institutionalization. The facts of institutionalization thus preclude any finding that residents are there voluntarily, or may leave at any time.

The legal decisions that emanate from right-to-treatment suits will inevitably shape future long-term-care policy. They reflect constitutional guarantees and embody a belief that the individual should receive care in a dignified, humane, and unrestricted manner.

Conclusions

The decision whether to mount a national program for the provision of long-term care is a serious one. It involves explicit acknowledgement of the role of the state as regards certain dependent groups, and acceptance of a commitment that may be costly and far-reaching, at a time when our available financial resources are contracting. The choices now facing us are difficult, influenced by legal imperatives, public attitudes, and economic and political constraints. Yet choices must be made.

How much we are willing to invest in the problem sets the broadest parameter of choice. Once that question is decided, resource allocation questions prevail. Should services be delivered to the old, the most impaired, or the poorest? How should factors such as income, assets, and informal supports be weighed in the service allocation decision? Responses to these questions will reflect society's values as regards human dignity, the quality of an extended life, and the quality of death. The second part of this essay has attempted to highlight the options open to policymakers as they decide who can and should be served under a national system of long-term care.

Recommendations

The policy puzzle of who should be served remains. The first part of this essay, a review of the populations-at-risk and potential demand for long-term-care services, concludes with several observations about the gaps remaining in current knowledge. These gaps, due to measurement problems, may never be filled. Thus data cannot answer the remaining questions.

Therefore the solution to the puzzle, as we have been suggesting, rests in the political arena wherein decisions of an economic, moral, and legal nature are weighed, one against the other. But the evidence presented does narrow somewhat the parameters of choice, suggesting the following set of recommendations.

1. Allocation decisions will be helped if the role of a public long-term-care system is clarified. The question of who should be served can be addressed only in the context of the kind of intervention that is desirable. We recommend that the role of services be twofold—protective and independence-enhancing. For those individuals whose physical and mental capacities are so diminished that self-care is impossible, the system should provide protective services that respect the inherent dignity of the individual while protecting him from harm. For others who have reduced capacity for self-care, a long-term-care system should provide, to the

greatest extent possible, services that rehabilitate and educate for self-maintenance.

2. Once this role has been established, we recommend that a long-term-care service system be available to all functionally disabled persons, regardless of age. The societal obligation rests upon compensation for the incapacity, not age, of the client.

3. Since the level of demand will be unrestricted but the level of services restricted, ability to pay will have to be considered as a rationing device. Since it can be presumed that the service needs of any functionally disabled person will prove costly, the tax system can compensate for these extraordinary costs through expanded credits and/or deductions. Disability insurance benefits can take into account special service needs of the individual, as can the Supplemental Security Income program. Services can also be supported through modest user fees, scaled to income.

4. Since it is generally seen as desirable to have informal support networks (family and friends) remain active service providers for the disabled individual, we recommend that, wherever possible, the family, not the individual, be the target of intervention.

5. Legal and ethical imperatives support the recommendation that the developing long-term-care system be the least restrictive possible. This recommendation does not lean toward a prohibition of institutions; rather, it supports the view that all services, institution- or community-based, respect the right of individual freedom from undue constraints.

Notes

1. The Medicare program, for example, is based upon the presumed inability of older persons to purchase hospital and medical insurance on the open market. Since the elderly are presumed to have higher medical care costs than younger groups, insurance is deemed desirable.

2. See, for example, U.S. Congress, Congressional Budget Office, *Long Term Care for the Elderly and Disabled* (1977), p. 16, wherein estimates of potential demand range from 5.5 to 9.9 million persons.

3. Ethel Shanas, *The Health of Older People: A Social Survey,* (Cambridge, Mass.: Harvard University Press, 1962); Ethel Shanas, Peter Townsend, D. Wedderburn, H. Friis, J. Milhoj, and J. Stehouwer, *Old People in Three Industrial Societies* (New York: Atherton, 1968); A. S. Harris, *Handicapped and Impaired in Great Britain* (London: Her Majesty's Stationery Office, 1971).

4. Robert Morris, "The Development of Parallel Services for the Elderly and Disabled," *Gerontologist* 14 (February 1974): 15.

5. U.S. Department of Health, Education, and Welfare, Social Security Administration, *First Findings of the 1972 Survey of the Disabled: General Characteristics* (Washington, D.C.: Government Printing Office, 1978), p. 1.

6. U.S. Department of Health, Education, and Welfare, National Center for Health Statistics, *State Estimates of Disability and Utilization of Medical Services: United States 1974–1976* (Washington, D.C.: Government Printing Office, 1977), p. 4.

7. Robert L. Clark and Joseph H. Spengler, "Changing Demography and Dependency Costs: The Implications of Future Dependency Ratios and Their Composition," in *Aging and Income*, ed. Barbara Rieman Herzog (New York: Human Sciences Press, 1978), p. 86.

8. Bernice L. Neugarten, "The Future and the Young-Old," *Gerontologist* 15, no. 1 (February 1975): 5, table 1.

9. U.S. Department of Commerce, Bureau of the Census, *One in Eleven: Handicapped Adults in America* (Washington, D.C.: President's Committee on Employment of the Handicapped, 1977), p. 2.

10. Aaron Krute and Mary Ellen Burdette, "1972 Survey of the Disabled and Nondisabled Adults: Chronic Disease, Injury, and Work Disability," *Social Security Bulletin* 41 (April 1978): 3.

11. R. C. Scheerenberger, *Deinstitutionalization and Institutional Reform* (Springfield, Ill.: Charles C. Thomas, 1976), p. 53.

12. G. Tarjan, S. Wright, R. Eyman, and R. Keeran, "Natural History of Mental Retardation: Some Aspects of Epidemiology," *American Journal of Mental Deficiency* 77 (1973): 372.

13. J. W. Singer, "It Isn't Easy to Cure the Ailments of the Disability Insurance Program," *National Journal*, May 6, 1978, pp. 715–19.

14. Council on Pediatric Practice, *Lengthening Shadows* (Evanston, Ill.: American Academy of Pediatrics, 1970), pp. 51–59.

15. National Foundation for the March of Dimes, *March of Dimes Facts*, 1979, p. 5.

16. Ibid., p. 7.

17. U.S. Department of Health, Education, and Welfare, National Center for Health Statistics, *Trends in "Prematurity," United States 1950–67* (Washington, D.C.: Government Printing Office, 1972), p. 2.

18. President's Commission on Mental Health, Volume I (Washington, D.C.: Government Printing Office, 1978), p. 4.

19. G. Klerman, "Better but Not Well: Social and Ethical Issues in the Deinstitutionalization of the Mentally Ill," *Schizophrenia Bulletin* 2 (1976): 580.

20. Judith Clark Turner and William J. TenHoor, "The NIMH Community Support Program: Pilot Approach to a Needed Social Reform," *Schizophrenia Bulletin* 4 (1978): 320.

21. See, for example, Edward A. Powers and Gordon L. Bultena, "Correspondence between Anticipated and Actual Uses of Public Services by the Aged," *Social Service Review* 48 (June 1974): 245–54.

22. M. Powell Lawton, "The Functional Assessment of Elderly People," *American Geriatrics Society* 19 (June 1971): 465–81.

23. John Kleh, "When to Institutionalize the Elderly," *Hospital Practice* (1977), pp. 121–29.

24. State of Illinois, Department of Aging, *Summary of the Major Findings of the Long Term Care Study* (Chicago: Booz, Allan and Hamilton, 1975).

25. Ronald Andersen and John F. Newman, "Societal and Individual Determinants of Medical Care Utilization in the United States," *Milbank Memorial Fund Quarterly* 51 (Winter 1973): 95–124.

26. William Pollak, *Expanding Health Benefits for the Elderly*, Volume I: *Long-Term Care* (Washington, D.C.: The Urban Institute, 1979), p. 19.

27. Powers and Bultena, "Correspondence between Anticipated and Actual Uses," pp. 245–54.

28. William Pollak, "Utilization of Alternative Care Settings by the Elderly," in *Com-

munity Planning for an Aging Society, ed. M. Powell Lawton, R. J. Newcomer, and Thomas O. Byerts (Stroudsburg, Pa.: Dowden, Hutchinson and Ross, 1976), p. 120.

29. Helena Z. Lopata, "Support Systems of Elderly Urbanites: Chicago of the 1970s," *Gerontologist* 15 (February 1975): 35–41.

30. See S. Brody, S. W. Poulshock, and C. Mosciocchi, "The Family Caring Unit: A Major Consideration in the Long-Term Care Support System," *Gerontologist* 18 (December 1978): 556–61; Marjorie Cantor, *Friends and Neighbors: An Overlooked Resource in the Informal Support System,* paper presented to the annual meeting of the Gerontological Society, November 1977; Ethel Shanas, "The Family as a Social Support System in Old Age," *Gerontologist* 19 (April 1979): 169–83; Amy Horowitz, *Families Who Care: A Study of Natural Support Systems of the Elderly,* paper presented at the annual meeting of the Gerontological Society, November 1978; U.S. Comptroller General, Report to Congress, *The Well-Being of Older People in Cleveland, Ohio* (Washington, D.C.: Government Printing Office, 1977).

31. Judith Treas, "Family Support Systems for the Aged: Some Social and Demographic Considerations," *Gerontologist* 17 (December 1977): 486–91.

32. Functional kin include a child or sibling whom the respondent sees at least monthly or is in phone contact with at least weekly, and include relatives who are living within the city and who are seen or heard from regularly.

33. Marjorie Cantor and J. Johnson, *The Informal Support System of the "Familyless" Elderly: Who Takes Over?* paper presented to the annual meeting of the Gerontological Society, November 1978.

34. Gerald M. Eggert, C. V. Granger, Robert Morris, and S. F. Pendleton, "Caring for the Patient with Long-Term Disability," *Geriatrics,* 1977, p. 110.

35. Pollak, "Utilization of Alternative Settings by the Elderly," p. 114.

36. U.S. Department of Labor, Bureau of Labor Statistics, *U.S. Working Women: A Databook* (Washington, D.C: Government Printing Office, 1977), p. 1.

37. P. C. Glick, "The Future Marital Status and Living Arrangements of the Elderly," *Gerontologist* 19 (June 1979): 308.

38. See the Mental Retardation Facilities and Mental Health Centers Construction Act of 1963, which encourages the development of community treatment centers; the Education for All Handicapped Children Act of 1975, which encourages "mainstreaming" of handicapped children; and the 1979 amendments to the Rehabilitation Act of 1973, which encourages the development of independent living centers for the disabled.

39. Harold L. Wilensky and Charles N. Lebeaux, *Industrial Society and Social Welfare* (New York: Free Press, 1965), p. xii.

40. Theodore R. Marmor, "The Congress: Medicare Politics and Policy," in *American Political Institutions and Public Policy,* ed. Allan P. Sindler (Boston: Little Brown, 1971), p. 19.

41. Irwin Garfinkel, untitled background paper for a conference on income-tested versus universal programs held at the University of Wisconsin, Institute for Research on Poverty, March 1979, p. 28.

42. U.S. Congress, Congressional Budget Office, *Long-Term Care for the Elderly and Disabled* (Washington, D.C.: Government Printing Office, 1977), p. 24.

43. D. Frankfather, M. Smith, and J. Capers, *Family Maintenance of the Disabled Elderly,* paper presented to the annual meeting of the American Orthopsychiatric Association, April 1979.

44. Brody, Poulshock, and Mosciocchi, "The Family Caring Unit," p. 560.

45. A. P. Fengler and N. Goodrich, "Wives of Elderly Disabled Men: The Hidden Patients," *Gerontologist* 19 (April 1979): 179.

46. J. R. A. Sanford, "Tolerance of Debility in Elderly Dependents by Supporters at Home: Its Significance for Hospital Practice," *British Medical Journal* 3 (1975): 471–73.

47. Edward Litwak, "Extended Kin Relations in an Industrial Democratic Society," in *Social Structure and the Family: Generational Problems,* ed. Ethel Shanas and Gordon Streib (New Jersey: Prentice-Hall, 1965).

48. Robert Moroney, *The Family and the State: Considerations for Social Policy* (London: Longman, 1976).

49. A. Lipman, "Ethics in Resource Allocation," in *Ethical Considerations in Long Term Care,* ed. W. J. Winston and A. J. Wilson III (St. Petersburg, Fla.: Eckerd College Gerontology Center, 1977), p. 76.

50. B. J. Diggs, "The Ethics of Providing for the Economic Well-Being of the Aging," in *Social Policy, Social Ethics and the Aging Society,* ed. B. L. Neugarten and R. J. Havighurst (Washington, D.C.: Government Printing Office, 1976), p. 57.

51. Eggert, Granger, Morris, and Pendleton, "Caring for the Patient with Long Term Disability," p. 115.

52. National Center for Law and the Handicapped, *The Right to Habilitation* (South Bend, Ind.: National Center for Law and the Handicapped, 1979), p. 5.

53. *Wyatt* v. *Stickney,* 325 F. Supp. 781 (M.D. Ala. 1971); 334 F. Supp. 1341 (M.D. Ala. 1971); 344 F. Supp. 373 (M.D. Ala. 1972); 344 F. Supp. 387 (M.D. Ala. 1972); *aff'd sub. nom., Wyat* v. *Aderholt,* 503 F. 2d 1305 (5th Cir. 1974), and *Welsh* v. *Likins,* 373 F. Supp. 487 (D. Minn. 1974), *aff'd in part and vacated and remanded in part,* 550 F. 2d 1122 (8th Cir. 1977).

54. *New York State Association for Retarded Children, Inc.,* v. *Rockefeller,* 357 F. Supp. 752, 764-5 (E.D.N.Y. 1973) and 393 F. Supp. 715, 718 (E.D.N.Y. 1975).

55. *Pennsylvania Association for Retarded Children* v. *Commonwealth of Pennsylvania,* 343 F. Supp. 279 (E.D. Pa. 1972).

56. *Horacek* v. *Exon,* 357 F. Supp. 71 (D. Neb. 1973) and No. 72-6-299 (D. Neb. 1975), and *Halderman* v. *Pennhurst State School and Hospital,* 446 F. Supp. 1295 (E.D. Pa. 1977).

5 Delivery of Services to Persons with Long-Term-Care Needs

James J. Callahan, Jr.

Introduction

The problem of delivery of long-term-care services is urgent although not new. The issue was treated very well by the Commission on Chronic Illness in 1956 in its volume, *Care of the Long-Term Patient*. The Commission noted the great difference between the acute patient and the chronic patient. In particular, it noted that the chronic patient needs simultaneous resolution of a number of problems, whereas the acute patient needs episodic solutions to consecutive problems. The volume discussed briefly a service delivery organization to meet the needs of the long-term patient. It noted:

> No single agency in any community can meet all the complex needs of the long-term patient; without some central organization concerned with those needs, gaps and overlaps in long-term care are almost inevitable. The task of such a central agency is formidable because of the wide range in needs of the long-term patient, the multiplicity of ways through which care is financed, conflicting interests and pressures, the existence of outmoded facilities and other factors. . . . Chronic illness is everyone's problem and, by the same token, no one's clear responsibility. . . . For the long-term patient, the absence of a single responsible agency is a major lack . . . the individual does not know where to turn.[1]

The document described comprehensively the range of services that such an individual requires. It noted also problems of financing, organization, resources, and manpower. Since 1956, great changes have taken place with respect to availability of funds, the number of agencies and organizations available, and the growth of manpower. What has not happened, however, has been the establishment of service delivery systems which meet long-term-care needs in an accountable and coordinated manner. As we discuss the long-term-care delivery options, it will be important to recognize this history and try to identify the factors which have prevented a resolution of the delivery system problems.

During the 1960s, long-term-care needs seemed to recede from the public consciousness. The passage of Medicare and Medicaid in 1965, and the problems associated with mounting those programs, seemed to draw attention away from long-term care. In addition, Medicaid pumped new money into nursing homes promising to improve care by medicalizing control. In the past few years, however, because of cost and service problems, attention has been refocused on the problem of long-term care. Between 1974 and 1978, a significant number of studies were conducted on long-term care which analyzed various options for its provision.[2] Many of the logical possibilities for delivery of services were covered in these papers. More recently, the University Health Policy Center, Brandeis University, has completed a set of long-term-care options papers for the Health Care Financing Administration.[3] These papers look at the options of long-term-care insurance, a disability allowance, block grants to the states, a case management system, a single long-term-care agency, and a social/health maintenance organization. Congress and the Executive Branch are now interested in testing new ideas for long-term care on a national basis and have provided $20 million in FY '80 for demonstrating "channeling" agencies.

The purpose of this paper is to bring together certain theoretical concepts and empirical findings as a basis for developing a national scheme for delivering services to persons with long-term-care needs. The paper will attempt to identify the dynamics of the present system(s) of delivery and how those dynamics might be harnessed to bring about changes that will improve life for persons with needs requiring long-term-care services. The paper will not propose a particular model but rather suggest an overall framework for policy decisions about long-term-care services.

The paper will define the problem, outline the goals of long-term care, describe salient characteristics of the long-term patient and long-term-care services, and present some theoretical considerations underlying the establishment and operation of delivery systems. It will also describe the present system of care, discuss some major problems in that system, and review past efforts of attempting to improve human service delivery systems. The paper will conclude with a discussion of possible policy approaches to the problem of long-term care.

The Problem of Long-Term Care

Problem definition is a useful first step to take if one hopes to change or improve a situation. One can arrive at a definition by saying what a thing is or what it is not. For the purposes of this paper, the problem of long-term care is not the problem of what to do about the rising cost and questionable quality of nursing homes. Rather, the problem to be addressed is how can this society develop a community-based, noninstitutional system for delivery of services to persons with long-term-care needs. While there may be a relationship between the two problems, the establishment of community-based, long-term-care delivery systems will not solve, in and of itself, the nursing home problem. The growth in expenditures for nursing homes is related only in part to patient demand. It reflects also the forces of inflation, regulations, private business speculation, and transfer of state institution costs to the federal government.

The growth in costs for nursing home care under the old public assistance titles, and subsequently under Medicaid, has been dramatic. Public nursing home expenditures increased from about $800 million in 1967 to about $3.628 billion in 1974 (see fig. 5.1). By the end of the next three-year period, 1974–77, under Medicaid, expenditures had reached $6.380 billion —an increase of $2.752 billion, or 75.85 percent.

Recipients however are not increasing at anywhere near the same rate as costs. According to a 1979 article in the *Social Security Bulletin,* the increase in total Medicaid expenditures during the 1974–75 period was attributed to the following: 58.0% to higher prices; 35.5% to changes in health practice such as increased technology and intensification of service; and only 6.0% to an increase in the number of recipients.[4] As can also be seen from figure 5.1, the increase in recipients has been at a much lower rate than the increase in costs. Although this 1979 article dealt with total Medicaid expenditures, it is not unreasonable to assume a similar pattern for a segment of the Medicaid program—nursing homes. Whether intensification of services reflects greater disability, improvement of care to an appropriate level, or overservice has not been determined.

The cost dimensions of the nursing home problem are immense. In 1977, as noted, a total of nearly $6.4 billion was spent under Medicare and Medicaid for nursing home care. Only $636 million was spent on home health care.[5] Nursing home charges have been growing at the rate of approximately 10 percent per year.[6] This means that in one year 10 percent inflation would require an additional $640 million for nursing homes without any increase in services. This inflation amount, $640 million, is more than the total spent on home health care by Medicare and Medicaid. It is obvious that the increase in cost for nursing homes is eating up potential funds for community-based programs. The nursing home problem will need to be attacked by controlling inappropriate intake into nursing homes, changing reimbursement methods, limiting supply, or some other steps. The point is that the development of a community-based long-term-care delivery system, in and of itself, will not solve the nursing home cost problem, and we should recognize that right from the start. This same conclusion was reached by Solem and Garrich in an evaluation of a community-based care project in the state of Washington. They noted:

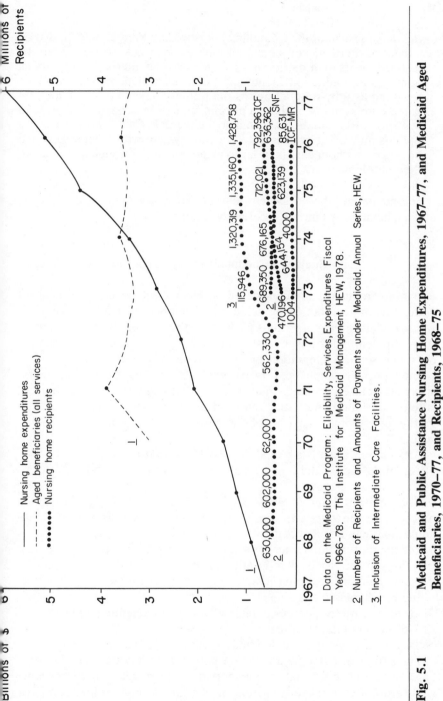

Billions of $

Millions of Recipients

—— Nursing home expenditures
----- Aged beneficiaries (all services)
•••• Nursing home recipients

1967 68 69 70 71 72 73 74 75 76 77

630,000 602,000 62,000
2

562,330

115,946
3

689,350 676,165 712,021 1,335,160 1,428,758
1,320,319

470,196 644,154 623,139
1004 4000
2

792,396 ICF
636,362 SNF
85,631 ICF-MR

1 Data on the Medicaid Program: Eligibility, Services, Expenditures Fiscal
   Year 1966-78. The Institute for Medicaid Management, HEW, 1978.

2 Numbers of Recipients and Amounts of Payments under Medicaid. Annual Series, HEW.

3 Inclusion of Intermediate Care Facilities.

Fig. 5.1   **Medicaid and Public Assistance Nursing Home Expenditures, 1967–77, and Medicaid Aged
Beneficiaries, 1970–77, and Recipients, 1968–75**

the major lesson of the Community-Based Care Project may be that an expanded network of community-based services will have to be justified on its own merits, not as a cost-saving alternative to nursing home care. Reduction in nursing home placement may have to be regarded as a by-product not as the primary objective of community-based care systems. Although per capita costs may be contained, total systems costs can be expected to increase because the increase in options may bring persons into the care system who otherwise would have gone without care in order to avoid notice or through ignorance of their entitlements.[7]

The community-based system may be necessary to a solution of the nursing home problem, but it certainly is not sufficient.

Goals of a Community Long-Term-Care System

Situations frequently are considered problems because unstated goals of various actors are not being achieved. Attempts are made at solutions where understanding of various goals is only presumed. In this case, there is great potential for misunderstanding and fruitless efforts. Commenting on social service integration projects, Agranoff noted: "At the risk of sounding overly simplistic, it is extremely crucial that service integration strategists closely ponder what and why they are integrating. Indeed, careful consideration of such questions from the very beginning of integration efforts may prove to be the singlemost important factor behind success."[8]

Articulating goals is a useful process because it makes various actors aware of their own and others' understanding of the situation and forms some basis for diaogue.

Goals exist at different levels of analysis. First-level goals relate to the outcomes of the long-term-care system for individuals. Five desired outcome goals can be identified:
1. Maximum functional independence at all times, even if there are limitations in activity or deterioration of function.
2. Rehabilitation, restoring him/her to some previous level of functioning which can be sustained.
3. Humane care for persons functionally and permanently dependent.
4. Utilization of the least restrictive environment.
5. Death with dignity for individuals in the dying process.

The particular outcome desired for particular individuals will differ according to the individual's characteristics and needs. These outcome goals are not mentioned frequently in the long-term-care literature, but they are nonetheless the justification for the existence of long-term-care services.

At a second level of analysis, goals are often stated:
1. To meet the medical/social needs of the entire long-term-care population.
2. To provide a coordinated comprehensive system of care.
3. To provide equal access to long-term-care services.
4. To reduce the cost of long-term-care services by more appropriate use of existing resources.

While there probably would be general agreement on these goals, there will be disagreement as to their relative priority.

The federal government is concerned primarily with costs and would like to develop alternatives to reduce inappropriate use of both hospitals and nursing homes. The point of view of state government is variable. Some states, like Massachusetts, California, and Pennsylvania, have moved ahead in the establishment of community support services. Other states have been reluctant and have actually retarded the growth of services by failing to develop adequate reimbursement policies for home health organizations and similar agencies. The elderly and their professional advocates are a strong constituency for expansion of home-based services. The Area Agencies on Aging and the National Council of Senior Citizens, for example, want to see an expansion of home-based services to reduce the dependence on nursing homes. A unique group concerned with the problem of long-term care is the disabled, whose achievements can be measured by the recent revisions during 1978 of the Rehabilitation Act. The disabled are perhaps the most radical of all the actors in the long-term-care arena, and are striving to redefine the tasks that need to be accomplished in long-term care. Long-term care is being translated into the language of civil rights, consumerism, and self help.[9]

At some point, somehow, agreement will have to be reached on at least a negotiated set of second-level goals for long-term care if any type of planned system of care is to be established. It is possible to "muddle through" with de facto goals. This appears, however, to be too limited an approach given the escalating costs and service demands. A more conscious planned approach to long-term care is required.

Context for Analysis of the Delivery of Long-Term-Care Services
Patient Characteristics

We noted earlier that the long-term-care patient, or disabled person, is different from the acute patient. His medical and/or personal needs exist for a period of many years and must be met more or less simultaneously by a variety of different providers. The individual must handle also the negative impact on his/her autonomy and decision making which may result from a period of long-term dependency. The disabled person will find that necessary absences from work may jeopardize a job. As the length of disability extends, exclusion and maximum benefit provisions of insurance policies take effect. Perhaps, most importantly, dependence on family members for personal care, transportation, and emotional support increases.

This family dimension is perhaps the least recognized yet most important element in planning a system to meet the needs of the disabled person.[10] While the individual may be the appropriate unit of eligibility for acute and/or episodic type services, a family or household may be a more appropriate unit for long-term community services to the disabled.

Describing the problems of children with chronic disabilities, Ireys noted:

> Still, a severe chronic handicap can impose great burdens: some children must cope with nagging pain, continued discomfort, a sense of being "different," dependent and perhaps unworthy; often they and their families must deal with very repetitive daily routines, financial burdens, stigma and pity from a well-intentioned society; or perhaps worst of all, diminished hopes. In other instances, handicaps are less disabling, though even here the sense and reality of being limited can threaten normal psychological growth and development. Furthermore, situations can change so that a family that was coping well somehow falters and never fully recovers.[11]

This description would apply also to the plight of many older disabled persons.

The unique characteristics of disabled persons and those caring for them point up the need not only for a special form of policy and service delivery, but also for special training and sensitivity on the part of staff dealing with long-term-care patients. Recognition of these unique patient characteristics must be built into the delivery system. Unfortunately, because of the nature of that system, this will be very difficult to accomplish.

Delivery System Characteristics

The most important characteristic of long-term-care services is that they are provided by so many human service subsystems. The long-term-care individual will draw upon the health subsystem, the housing subsystem, the income maintenance subsystem, the educational subsystem, the employment subsystem, and the personal social service subsystem to find the full range of services he requires. We refer to this as the *intersystem concept,* and it is very important because it identifies the sectors where linkages may be required to meet needs of the disabled person.

A system can be conceived of as a set of interrelated parts or components such that the behavior of components affect one another. The components interact within an environment with exchange taking place across system boundaries. A system may have very clearly defined boundaries and easily identifiable components. A system, however, may have ill-defined boundaries with components that are difficult to observe. The key idea is that certain elements tend to cluster and interact together within certain boundaries.

It is possible to identify subsystems in the human services field even though boundaries may not be precisely defined or centers of system control be observable. Sets of activities, interests, professions, and funding sources that cluster together comprise a subsystem. A comparison between the health subsystem and the housing subsystem will serve to illustrate the point.

Subsystem Characteristic	Health	Housing
Prime activity	care of patients	construction of buildings
Professions	physicians, nurses, therapists	architects, builders, bankers
Funding sources	third parties, government (HEW)	banks, government (HUD)

An ideology or thought structure, of necessity, accompanies activities performed within a subsystem and shapes the decisions made about disabled people. For example, persons entering the health system are "patients," while those going into public housing are "tenants." There are expectations for certain forms of behavior on the part of both subsystem personnel and disabled individuals themselves. Individual needs get met to the extent that they fit the needs of the various subsystems.[12]

Because the disabled person partakes of these different subsystems, a need for case coordination and subsystem linkages is presumed to exist. While this is a reasonable assumption with many case examples to support it, the number of persons requiring case coordination is not known, nor are the nature and extent of required linkages among the subsystems. Data will be needed in both areas as the intersystem concept is refined.

A second important characteristc of long-term services is that one of the subsystems of most importance to the disabled person, namely, the personal social service subsystem, is poorly organized and barely exists as a system. This is a real problem because many of the services most needed are those of a personal social service nature. The National Conference on Social Welfare, in its 1977 report, "The Future for Social Services in the United States,"[13] and the American Public Welfare Association, in a report of its Policy Committee on Social Services,[14] have pointed up the need to integrate and coordinate social services through a personal social service system independent of the subsystems described above. Both of these groups would see the personal social service system as the entry point and case manager for persons with long-term-care needs. Currently, there is competition among the public social service sector, Area Agencies on Aging, mental health system, developmental disabilities system, and so forth. Whether the personal social services system can be organized in the short-term is very unlikely.

A third characteristic of the present service system is that in many instances the long-term-care individual is *marginal* to the service providers upon which he/she depends. For example, income maintenance workers are concerned with establishing eligibility for income assistance, and not with the other related concerns of the disabled person, such as housing or transportaion. Health services are concerned primarily with the acute needs or episodes faced by a long-term-care individual and not with the prior or subsequent living arrangements that may influence that health problem. The majority of the organizations upon which the disabled person is dependent serve mostly those who do not have long-term-care needs. This includes the income maintenance agencies and hospitals as already mentioned, but also groups such as senior citizen centers that direct their attention to the well elderly. The implication is that the attention that the disabled individual requires may not be given, and that the necessary linkages that may have to be made will be overlooked. In addition, some of the agenices that have disabled individuals as their major clients tend to be themselves marginal to the health and social service system. For example, nursing homes are seen as standing more or less outside of the "respected" agencies. Homemaker agencies are new to the scene, as are centers for independent living. This marginality affects their ability to impact on the broader systems on behalf of their clients.

There are four identifiable sectors which serve as subgroups of the long-term-care population. These sectors are: (1) the child sector which would include parents, school system, child welfare agencies, and teaching hospitals for the handicapped child;[15] (2) the young adult sector, which would include the vocational rehabilitation agency, the specialized services for the handicapped such as the independent living centers, families, and peers; (3) the disabled adult sector, which would include the vocational rehabilitation agency, the spouse, and perhaps the parents of the adult; (4) the elderly sector, which would include Area Agencies on

Aging, senior citizen centers, specialized day care programs, meal programs, and the siblings and children of the elderly. A fifth sector, which does not share the characteristics of the others, is the community mental health system, which appears to be developing its own coordinated comprehensive, isolated system. The existence of these different sectors suggests that we ought not to try to establish one system that would incorporate the total picture. This will be discussed later in this paper.

Patterns of Long-Term-Care Services

The range of services required by persons with long-term-care needs is impressive. Nearly every human service sector provides a service needed at least some time by some individuals. There are many lists of required services available in the literature. The National Conference of Social Welfare categorizes over seventy long-term-care resources and services under three general headings:[16]
1. *Intramural:* 24-hour residential services for long-term/intermittent/ acute treatment.
2. *Intermediate:* nonresidential, fewer than 24 hours; person goes to agency or service locale.
3. *Extramural:* Services are provided at the site of the problem, i.e., home, school, by an individual worker or practitioner and/or agency personnel.

The American Public Welfare Association identified 12 categories of services needed by persons with long-term-care needs.[17] Most volumes dealing with long-term care have their own list of services. Since many of the lists span the range of human services, they are not very useful for identifying the type, amount, and frequency most required by long-term individuals. Perhaps more important, they do not set priorities. An attempt has been made, however, to identify a minimum set of nonacute medical services that would be required by the long-term-care individual.[18] The list reflects the judgment of a number of experts in the field of long-term care. These services are: case management, chore services, home-delivered meals, home health aide, homemaker assistance, physical therapy, protective services, skilled nursing, telephone reassurance/daily checking, transportation, supervised living arrangements, information and referral services, emergency mental health support, and nursing home care.

While some of the identified services are provided individually, they are usually considered part of a delivery system. Most experts would agree that, ideally, the services of the long-term-care delivery system should be available, accessible, and acceptable. They also should be comprehensive, continuous, and coordinated. These admittedly general criteria reflect an ideal state which does not exist. Where do we now stand, however, in respect to meeting these criteria? We really do not know objectively, and expert opinion would differ. The fact is, however, that citizens are receiving long-term-care services and depending on public and private expenditures to a significant degree.

The largest amount of long-term caring activity is provided by family members in the home. Most of this may be appropriate, and much may be given without any significant burden on the family. On the other hand, if much of this care is to varying degrees inappropriate and/or burdensome, families would benefit from community-based resources. Accurate measures of these situations do not now exist.

Data are available, however, for community-based services. Nursing homes currently house about 1.3 million people. Some of these individuals do not belong in nursing homes, but by any estimate at least 700,000–800,000 do require a residential setting with professional nursing care on a twenty-four-hour basis.[19] Home health agencies are serving over 700,000 individuals per year. Many would argue that this is too low a number, but few would argue that much of it is inappropriate. In addition to health services, on a yearly basis nearly 3 million individuals are receiving congregate meals; over 2 million are receiving social services under Title XX; and over 11 million are being served under Title III of the Older Americans Act.[20] Approximately 1.8 million days of adult day care were delivered to older persons in 1977.[21] Services are provided by some 18,000–20,000 nursing homes, 614 long-term hospitals, 6,600 general hospitals, over 2,100 home health agencies, 600 Area Agencies on Aging, over 2,000 nutrition sites, and tens of thousands of local agencies of various types. The services are provided in over fifty states plus the territories. Where this amount of delivered service would locate us with respect to the ideal criteria is not known, but we should presume that we are well above zero.

The delivery of these services at the community level is usually complex. Callahan, in a study of social services in the Worcester, Massachusetts, area, identified over 178 agencies serving a population of about 250,000.[22] Fifty-seven of them offered information and referral services and 50 provided personal counseling. On the other hand, only one agency offered foster home care for adults. Many of the agencies were small, with 51 percent having budgets under $100,000. An interesting finding from the point of view of examining federal policy was that 22 percent of the voluntary agencies had federal funds as their *major* source of income.

Experience with Title XX gives some idea of how a federal social service program might affect the local community. This federal program gives considerable leeway to the states to define problems and services, to set eligibility levels, and to focus services on specific geographic areas.

Few, if any, of the states provide identical services. Some states provide as few as four; others as many as thirty. Definitions of the services vary from state to state. In addition, there is variation in eligibility criteria. Six states provide all of their services to a specified level of income; 39 states vary eligibility by service; 38 states vary eligibility by category and individual; 9 states vary eligibility by geographic area; and 22 states use group eligibility. None of these categories is mutually exclusive, so that one finds variation within variation.[23] Certainly it would be possible for the federal government to standardize eligibility criteria as well as to standardize a set of services for the long-term care individual. It is not clear, however, that such a standardized approach to these problems would be as good as the pattern of variation that exists under Title XX. One could argue that the local determination of eligibility and services takes into account the existence of cultural and social factors as well as other program resources that may not be known to the federal government. The real challenge will be to design a system that ensures some level of national equity and, at the same time, builds on the unique foundation of the local service system.

Community Delivery Systems

To this point we have identified the general problem of long-term care, discussed goals, and identified the unique aspects of persons with long-term-care needs and of the subsystems which serve them. The actual delivery of services to disabled persons takes place within a given geographic location, by particular providers under specific conditions. In other words, receipt of services occurs within a specific community network of service.

The nature of the structures and processes of local community networks will have a major impact in shaping the delivery of long-term-care services. These local community networks have been referred to as the interorganizational field, and a large body of literature on them is available. One of the first analyses was that of Sol Levine and Paul E. White, focusing on the concept of exchange.[24] The authors attempted to explain interorganizational behavior as a form of exchange involving three main elements: clients, labor services, and resources other than labor services. Litwak and Hylton attempted to explain interorganizational behavior in terms of organizational interdependence, the level of organizational awareness, standardization of organization activities, and the number of organizations in the field.[25] While both these analyses focused on the interaction of one agency with another, a third, that of Warren, examined the behavior of the total interorganizational field as a system.[26]

Warren studied the behavior of community decision organizations (Model Cities agencies, Community Action agencies, school systems, health and welfare planning councils, mental health planning agencies) in nine cities. He noted that while coordinative and conflict activity occurred among the individual agencies, little real change or innovation took place. Coordination and conflict activities appear as epiphenomena in a situation where the total effect of activity is to maintain the local system of arrangements. According to Warren, the local communities are characterized by an institutional thought structure which limits options and gives meaning only to particular items of data while excluding others:

> Perhaps the most important global aspect of the interorganizational field is this basic agreement on definitions of social reality and social problems, respective agency domains, and ground rules for interaction, within which interaction is limited both in frequency and in the scope of issues involved. In this framework, the basic problems of the city are seldom addressed.[27]

Lest this discussion appear too theoretical, it should be noted that this finding of Warren's apparently was confirmed by Hainline and Lindsey in an analysis of aging services networks in six cities.[28] The authors focused on the problems that area agencies face in implementing their policies and the fact that many of these problems result from the agencies' need to integrate themselves into the communities in which they are located. The authors state: "Although our analysis of service networks indicates considerable variation in service networks among communities, we have also discovered evidence of commonality. An ordered system of interdependency occurs in all communities."[29]

Mechanic discusses the interorganizational linking process in terms of the principle of reciprocity. He notes how these links serve as a survival base for the existing community pattern. He states: "Any continuing attempt to challenge such community relationships, to undermine the power of particular community groups, or to support one community group against others—whatever the merits of the case—will soon lead those responsible to be labelled as troublemakers and deviants. If they manage to survive at all, they will soon find it difficult to sustain sufficient cooperation to do their jobs."[30]

These theoretical points have been validated in actual experiments and demonstrations which attempted to coordinate and integrate a local service system. Failures of federal attempts to pull together services on behalf of some particular client group are noteworthy. Both the Community Action Program and the Model Cities Program were aimed at imposing a structure of coordination and integration. While there were certainly benefits from these efforts, and a good deal of learning, neither program exists as a continuing vehicle of coordination and social change.

Morris and Lescohier examined nine studies that reviewed approximately one hundred state and local service integration efforts.[31] Included were those supported by HEW as prototypes for the Allied Services Act and as part of the Services Integration Target of Opportunity projects. Success in creating permanent structures and processes of coordination and integration appears to be nonexistent except for some specialized programs in rural areas operated by state government. Given that rural areas frequently lack services, success of these projects may reflect the impact of new resources rather than the coordination and integration of existing providers. Very few projects funded under these programs continue to exist.[32]

Aiken, et al., examined five case studies of coordinated services for the mentally retarded.[33] None of these projects accomplished all that was intended of it. An insufficient supply of the needed services, multiplicity of political jurisdictions and organizations, and lack of resources made "success" impossible.

More focused projects, and those of lesser scope, have not fared much better. What has been referred to as "the most carefully conceived and executed deinstitutionalization project yet undertaken in this country" did not survive more than two years.[34] The Community Life Association of Hartford, Connecticut, which was to be a model of integrated neighborhood service delivery, ended after three years despite the support of the Greater Hartford Process, Inc., which represented both the public and the business power structure of Hartford.[35] Although many of these projects were of a "demonstration" nature and designed mainly to provide knowledge, a frequent expectation was that they would become permanent.

That these failings occurred may be discouraging, but they should not be a surprise to persons familiar with interorganizational theory and research. Steinberg has pointed out numerous lessons from the past hundred years of social welfare history which are relevant to today's problems of service delivery.[36] Some of the more important lessons learned are as follows:

1. No one program model suits all communities.
2. The majority of users of innovative multipurpose or case coordination projects are *not* the at-risk population for which that particular program was designed.
3. The agency which coordinates other agencies should not operate direct services.
4. Coordination is very expensive, as well as difficult. Don't try to coordinate too many agencies at once.

5. Public/voluntary agency funding contracts can work, but successful coordination requires moderate stress.
6. Consumer and community involvement is difficult, takes time, and is a two-edged sword. Different degrees of community control are indicated for different kinds of objectives.
7. Co-location does not equal coordination. Unification of different services, under one administration, does not guarantee coordination.
8. Authority helps but does not guarantee coordination. Cooperative models rarely succeed.
9. Accountability mechanisms are hellish to install and maintain, but can be productive in time.
10. A coordination system should be evolutionary and cumulative.
11. The potential efficiency and effectiveness of a coordination program cannot be evaluated during the first and second years. (This does not preclude performance monitoring and documenting the experience and the rate of progress.)
12. The leader of a coordination project must be a super being with optimum political skills, administrative competence, missionary fervor and familiarity with the entire range of professional interventions and management techniques. In addition, the leader must, during the early phases of the new project, be primarily process-oriented and, in later phases, be primarily task-oriented.
13. At all levels of coordination, it is crucial that there be frequent and genuine interpersonal contact between representatives of agencies who are essential to the program's success.

These points should be considered as suggestive and instructive, not as normative design features of a delivery system. For example, item 3 which excludes direct service by a coordinating agency has long been an element of practice wisdom, but has not been scientifically proven as valid in all situations. Point 12 which notes the need for "super beings" to lead a coordination project raises some interesting questions. Are coordination projects setting themselves up for failure if they are designed for super beings when the supply of super beings apparently is so limited? Do super beings really exist or are these just the people who happen to be part of a program that is lucky enough to succeed? Modest approaches to coordination that can be managed by mere mortals may be more appropriate. Program implementation structures, matrix management, and networking may offer alternative approaches.[37]

What are the implications of these theoretical considerations and empirical findings for the establishment of long-term-care services in communities? Perhaps the major conclusion is that the success of any national long-term-care program will be shaped by the nature of the interorganizational field and organizational relationships in particular communities.

Although direct funding from Washington would provide a local long-term-care agency with considerable purchasing power, it is probable that the agency would be forced to purchase from the existing field of services and organizations. This is particularly true given our discussion above of the intersystem and the fact that many of the agencies upon which the long-term-care individual is dependent serve a much broader clientele and may be able to adopt a "take it or leave it" attitude. While the input of federal funds might make it possible to stimulate the creation of additional new organizations, one could expect considerable effort by the local community either to prevent, to blunt, or to repel such a development.[38] Certainly a massive federal intervention with additional dollars that could set up a competing system could be relatively free of the local interorganizational field. This type of intervention on a national basis, however, is doubtful, and a more limited program should be anticipated.

While we have made it clear that the local system of arrangements and interactions serves to contain change within certain boundaries, the locality itself is severely limited by vertical constraints imposed by state, federal, and national forces. The relationship of the vertical and horizontal dimensions of a community have been described in great detail by Warren.[39] Recently, Sydney Gardner discussed the limitation on policy space available to local human services managers. He listed eleven factors that constrict flexibility of local human service managers.[40]

1. The workings of the national economy as it affects the resources available to local policy makers.
2. The deliberate results of national policy such as a support for categorical grants or regulatory policies requiring environmental impact statements.
3. The inadvertent effects of national policy such as a support for suburbanization which resulted from the Highway Act in the tax structure.
4. The role of state government.
5. The role of public opinion and constraining local actors.
6. The views of outside political actors themselves, unions, interest groups and individual citizens.
7. Geography of the city and region (e.g., the degree to which the city's boundaries incorporate or are separate from the metropolitan economy, allowing linkage of local dollars outside the locality itself and in the region).
8. Demography since the make-up of the city's populations constrains its policy.
9. The city's own resources in light of both actual fiscal strength and its taxpayers' perceptions of their tax burdens.
10. Time as a constraint on short-range policymaking.
11. Judicial decisions as they set the legal boundaries of local policy.

In summary, any local system of service delivery to persons with
long-term-care needs will confront the existing distribution and interaction of power and interest. These local phenomena reflect the workings of
national and state forces, and these forces can be modified by action at the
national and state levels. For example, a national decision to abolish the
PSRO or HSA programs would remove a couple of actors from the local
scene. This points up the need to take action at all levels of government if
an effective local system of delivery is to be created.

Potential Sources of Change

The previous section described forces operating at the local level that
make it difficult to achieve the ends of purposeful federal intervention.
The limit imposed on local policy options by state and federal action was
also noted. The fact that these different levels are apt to frustrate each
other's goals does not mean that changes are not occurring which may be
beneficial to disabled people; nor are new delivery models ruled out. Life
goes on despite federal/local incompatibilities or inaction. In fact, some
community actors are clever enough to exploit this situation in their own
behalf. In the arena of long-term care, for instance, Medicare, Medicaid,
and Title XX are being utilized—sometimes very creatively.

A wide variety of services are being provided, will continue to be provided, and, in all probability, will expand. Although system maintenance
relationships within the organizational field may be relatively stable,
changes are occurring all the time. It is important to try to identify real
sources of change and to utilize them for the benefit of disabled people.
Four sources of change I consider important are:

1. *Expansion in the number of elderly and disabled.* The number of
elderly persons is increasing every year and, as a result, there will be
more pressure on the system to respond to their needs. The same is true of
the disabled population, although it is increasing at a slower rate than that
of the elderly. The existence of a large pool of individuals requiring service will put pressure on the system to deliver that service. Demographics
is a hard variable that accounts for much social change.[41]

2. *Expansion of the manpower pool of care providers.* It is now apparent that we may end up with an oversupply of physicians. It seems that we
have an oversupply of social workers, at least from the number of re-
sumés that I receive. A large number of universities are training both
undergraduate and graduate students in the area of gerontology. All of
these individuals are, or will be, out on the job market seeking jobs, and
this pressure of job seekers may have the effect of increasing the number
of jobs and funds available in gerontology and long-term care. White and

Gates have noted that one of the most important factors moving the United States toward a services economy is the employment needs of the middle class:[42] "Hence we choose to create services employment—most of which in the public sector is intended to alleviate 'social problems'— which appears more and more to have little true effect except to distribute various forms of personal income (in differential amounts) to service professionals and their clients."[43]

3. *The professional dynamic.* Miller has noted that professions are composed of competing subgroups each trying to attain dominance in the profession.[44] To achieve this dominance, subgroups will attempt to find important issues or areas of practice which they can use as a base for movement to the elite strata of the profession. This is beginning to show up in the area of medicine where "geriatrics" has become legitimated and many medical schools are beginning to develop specialties in this area. One also finds examples of geriatric nursing and specializations in gerontology in a variety of professional schools.

4. New consciousness on the part of client groups. In the first part of the paper, we noted the move by the severely disabled to obtain a reorientation of the caring system to their definition of their needs. Similar pressure is being exerted by elderly groups in combination with certain professional "elites" seeking to further their professional careers. This combination of client consciousness and professional dynamism should result in more responsive and appropriate service for the long-term-care patient. While providers will continue to provide what they are trained to provide, consumers should receive at least half-a-loaf of the bargain they strike with the professionals. If client groups are able to sustain themselves as citizen organizations, a greater degree of change will be brought about.

The four factors listed should have an impact on increasing the amount of financing for long-term-care services. Funds will flow differentially into areas and programs supported by professionals and citizens. The result will be some change and, we hope, an improvement in the life of the long-term-care individual. Earlier the paper noted the existence of identifiable sectors which reflect certain subgroups of the long-term-care population. These were identified as the child sector, the young adult sector, the disabled adult sector, the elderly sector, and the mental health sector. Table 5.1 attempts to relate these subsectors of the long-term-care population with the sources of change in the long-term-care field. This is done to help predict where and what type of change might take place and to identify potential loci of intervention for federal and state governments. The degree to which improvement occurs and its rate will depend upon many factors. At the present time, however, I do not see much more than incremental improvements along directions already agreed to by those

**Table 5.1   Sources of Change and Sectors of Service in
                  Long-Term Care**

Demography	Manpower Growth	Professional Dynamics	Client Consciousness
Child			
Large population getting smaller both absolutely and proportionally	Apparently still growing. Huge education sector in existence	Special education rising within the profession	Parent groups strong. Education of the Handicapped Act
Handicapped young adult			
Small population not growing fast	Growing. Expansion area for universities	Work with handicapped becoming more legitimate	Very high. New Rehabilitation Amendment
Disabled adult			
Moderately large, moderate increase	Unknown. May not be large	Unknown. Apparently not important	Not very visible
Elderly			
Moderate population growing absolutely and proportionally	Expanding substantially	Many professional subgroups moving into this area	Very high. Many organized interest groups

concerned with long-term care (e.g., deinstitutionalization, participation of clients in decision making, coordinated approaches to care).

Selected Models of Long-Term-Care Service Delivery

Policy approaches are difficult enough to develop, but their development becomes even more difficult in the absence of agreement about goals. It is not clear, for example, whether the federal government wishes to reduce expenditures in long-term care, expand services to the unserved, or both. Whatever the goal, there are at least two basic approaches which could be taken:
1. Develop an ideal delivery model to be adopted by all jurisdictions around the country.

2. Build on the positive elements of the existing mechanisms through a planned set of incremental changes.

Certainly, adoption of an "ideal" model around the country is not without merits. It would provide some national level of equity; it would provide comparable data for program planning and evaluation; and it would reflect a national attempt to handle the problem of service delivery for the long-term individual. Its main drawback is the infeasibility both of getting it enacted at a national level and of implementing it at the local level. Clearly a more incremental and expedient approach is called for. Frieden has remarked in connection with service integration efforts: "In program after program, demands for perfect equity, greater innovation, and more efficient use of resources were more destructive than helpful. They diverted the attention of administrators from goals that were simpler but more achievable, such as delivering resources to people in genuine need."[45]

Different incremental-type approaches have been identified. Morris and Lescohier, after their review of service integration projects, proposed two limited models which they believe may be feasible.[46]

1. The most promising future lies in the direction of a *delimited coordination* which relies upon the following components: (a) reinforcing the existing loose network of service providers through improved information and referral mechanisms; (b) a limited external control over the flow of resources to this network, by empowering a central unit to reserve a marginal proportion of the total flow of funds; (c) the reserved funds kept within the authority of the central control be used to fill gaps and to induce agencies to reduce their rates of client rejection; (d) the development of a capability at the central control level to identify and monitor client reject patterns and service gaps.
2. The alternative model of limited *integration* would seem to be feasible for a limited number of publicly administered social services now scattered in several large bureaucracies with extensive missions. Some of these social services could be merged under a unitary administration to carry out limited functions clearly in the domain of public service and complementary to the large bureaucracies from which they are drawn.

Aiken, et al., evaluated five different models.[47] They distinguished between three levels of coordination: professional level, program level, and institutional level. Resources are best coordinated at the institutional level, programs at the program level, clients at the professional level, and information at all three. This notion of different levels for coordination of different activities was noted also by Callahan in his discussion of the single long-term care agency,[48] and by Agranoff.[49] Aiken's, Callahan's, and Agranoff's levels line up as follows:

	Aiken	Callahan	Agranoff
Level 1	Institutional	System management	Policy
Level 2	Managerial	Operational management	Agency/Program
Level 3	Professional	Patient	Client/Service

While there are some differences, all three authors note that different levels of organization are required for the coordination of different activities. Aiken has attempted to evaluate the effectiveness of different models to coordinate specific elements (table 5.2).

Both Pollak and Callahan have examined models of a single agency to be the focal point of care for the long-term individual.[50] Callahan broke down the various functions of such an agency and indicated how those functions could be packaged differently to meet various objectives and/or local situations (table 5.3). Pollak identified and evaluated four models. He assumed a situation where federal funding sources were combined, resource authorization centralized, and consumers rather than producers subsidized. The four models are:

1. *Extreme centralization*—a single agency does patient assessment, service authorization, case management, and actual production of services.
2. *Moderate centralization*—a single agency does patient assessment authorization and case management, but services are purchased.
3. *Decentralization I*—a single agency does patient assessment and authorization, but case management and services are provided by other agencies.
4. *Decentralization II*—same as decentralization I, except that case management and production of service would be done, in most cases, by a single agency.

There are three other models worth thinking about. They are:
1. The single federal agency model
2. The public social service model
3. The Association of Users model

The single federal agency model would involve the establishment of an agency similar to the Veterans Administration or the Social Security Administration, with offices all over the country. To minimize dependence on local service systems, it could provide—like the V.A.—most services under its own auspice. On the other hand, it could serve merely a case

Table 5.2	Kinds of Service Delivery Structures and Elements to be Coordinated		
Type or Organizational Structure or Form			
Information[a]	Clients	Programs	Resources
Single organization with some services for a multiproblem client			
Equally effective	Ineffective	Ineffective	Ineffective
Single organization with all services for a single multiproblem client			
Equally effective	Most effective[b] or	Most effective[b]	Less effective
Single organization with wide range of services for all clients			
Equally effective	Most effective[c] or	Most effective[c]	Less effective
Coalition of organizations for a single multiproblem client			
Equally effective	Less effective	Most effective	Less effective
Community board			
Equally effective	Less effective	Less effective	Most effective

[a]Each form is likely to be as effective for information coordination as for coordination of the element it is most effective with.
[b]A single specialized organization—one handling all multiproblem clients of a particular kind —can coordinate clients or programs but not both equally effectively.
[c]A single organization designed to handle all clients needing physical, psychological, and social services can handle coordination of clients or of programs but not both equally effectively.

management role. Such a national organization is probably not feasible at the present time, but it is a conceivable model.

The public social service model is similar to that promoted by the National Conference of Social Welfare and the American Public Welfare Association (see above). Its features would include the following:

1. The local delivery unit would be the point of access (centrally or at out-stations) to all the long-term-care services.

2. The local delivery unit would provide the full range of case management activities.

3. All service resources which are publicly funded, whether purchased or agency provided, should reside in a pool or inventory available for use in individual case plans in accordance with the plan developed between case manager and client.

4. Each local public service delivery unit should have a certain amount

Table 5.3	Long-Term-Care System Array of Functions		
System Management			
Financing A1			
Planning B1	System Development B2	System Control B3	Evaluation B4
Operational Management			
Advocacy C1	Information System C2	Coordination C3	Quality Control C4
Payment of Bills C5			
Patient Management			
Outreach D1	Entry D2	Assessment & Care Planning D3	Eligibility Certification D4
Case Management D5	Service Delivery D6	Patient Information D7	Quality Control D8

of authority to choose the mix, quantity, and providers of services within its territory of responsibility, subject to existing regulations and possible requirements to use other public services if they are available.

The Association of Users model would involve the creation of nonprofit organizations of users (children and their parents, elderly, handicapped). One all-inclusive, or two or three specialized, organizations would be created in each jurisdiction. These organizations would recruit a certain number of members of the designated population group and, once having reached a certain size (10%–15% of target group), would be recognized by the federal government through a process similar to that of recognizing PSRO, HSA, or HMO but with many fewer criteria. The organization would receive a certain sum per member from the federal government, could charge minimal dues, and could solicit contributions. The function of these groups would be to negotiate packages of services with local providers, provide case management services for members unable to do so on their own, and work with federal and state governments to eliminate red tape and eligibility barriers. Other functions might be added, if feasible. The groups would not control the actual payment for service, but could control the flow of patients who were members. This would shift some power from providers to user groups, and should have the effect of making service somewhat more responsive to consumer needs. This arrangement would not help control costs except by making services more responsive and presumably less institutionally oriented. Government would still have to allocate total resources, but an additional formal voice would be added to that process.

This chapter has reviewed different models of service integration/delivery that have been proposed by experts in the field of long-term care. Most of the expert wisdom seems to advise a selective and incremental approach to change, which recognizes local variation, rather than a radical national solution to the problems of long-term care.

Ishizaki, Gottesman, and MacBride, for example, call for an incremental approach based on an assessment of local conditions: "A good system can only be fashioned if it comes from an assessment of the service-delivery reality in the community it serves. The first step in setting up service management is an assessment of that reality."[51]

A Proposed Policy Approach to Long-Term Care

The previous sections of this paper analyzed the problem of long-term care. This section attempts to use that analysis as at least a partial base for developing a policy approach to long-term care. It is, however, difficult to make a direct translation from the analysis to a suggested policy. A policy approach draws not only upon the analysis of the problem but also on ideological perspectives, assessment of political realities, personal judgments, and similar factors. The proposed policy approach, therefore, should be judged on the basis of not just the previous analysis, but also the reader's broader perspective on social policy informed by this analysis.

Critical Assumptions

There are certain assumptions upon which the policy proposal will be based:

1. At the local delivery level many things are happening now to improve the lot of the long-term-care individual. The various client sectors are taking advantage of existing programs, including Medicare, Medicaid, Title XX, and state-funded programs, to bring about an improvement in services they require. These sectors will look upon any federal intervention as an opportunity to expand what they are doing within their understanding of their interest. Even in the absence of a federal intervention, these various forces will continue to expand the amount of activity going on in the long-term-care area.

2. It is to the benefit of the federal government to maintain the interest and concern in long-term care of the various local actors. If the federal government wants to improve the lot of patients with long-term-care

needs, it is very important that those groups now involved maintain their interest and contribution—particularly in light of the intersystem nature of the service networks.

3. It is in the interest of the federal government to have local financial resources now available to the long-term-care population not only maintained, but also expanded.

4. Any federal effort must target itself to each subset of problems in the long-term-care field; specifically, it must distinguish between the problem of excessive nursing home costs and utilization and the need to develop a community-based care system.

Policy Proposal

The federal government should take leadership in developing national goals and policy for long-term care. The following steps should be taken:

1. Congress should create a joint House-Senate committee or subcommittee on long-term care to review the provisions of all existing legislation (health, social service, special education) for the purpose of eliminating barriers to service integration and creating legislative linkages.

Rationale. The array of programs operating at the local level reflects the categorical nature of much of the legislation which created and funds these programs. Change at the very top is needed if complexity is to be reduced at the lower levels. Attempts to get Congress to simplify or combine categorical programs have not been very successful. In fact, one might argue that while categories create certain barriers to coordination, they serve to make more resources available because they provide a focal point around which to organize a constituency. This issue, however, at least should be reviewed and barriers eliminated that will not jeopardize constituent interests.

2. The executive branch should establish, at the highest level, a Cabinet Interdepartmental Task Force to consolidate information on all federal programs (housing, health, etc.) affecting long-term care and to develop a plan for coordinating federal programs.

Rationale. The intersystem concept highlights the dependency of the disabled person on different subsystems. The federal government is funding and regulating many of the organizations within these subsystems. In addition, it is defining eligibility for programs affecting disabled persons. Because of the cost of long-term care and the coming impact of demographic change, the federal government should be looking at its total commitment in this area and doing what it can to improve performance. Another task force is not the ultimate answer, but it could make long-term care more salient in the public agenda.

3. As part of the Interdepartmental Task Force, a national nursing home planning project should be established within DHEW to review the national nursing home situation, including needs, costs, financing, and reimbursement. The output of this task force should be a national nursing home policy dealing with the respective roles of the federal government, the states, and the private sector.

As part of that policy, the federal government could establish a program to restrict access to nursing homes. PSROs would have their authority extended to include preadmission review for publicly aided patients to both skilled and intermediate care facilities. The PSRO screening unit would include a physician, nurse, social worker, and consumer. The purpose of this screening would be to act as a "barrier" to unnecessary placement in nursing homes. The PSRO screening unit would have absolutely no responsibility for coming up with an alternative placement for a case that it rejected. The responsibility for finding alternative resources and programs would lie with the agency (e.g., hospital, home health agency) or the individual (self, family) who made the referral. It is recognized, however, that in some instances other alternatives will not be available and that the nursing home will be the only recourse even though the individual does not require the range of services available in that setting. In such an event, a mechanism for appeal would exist and the individual could be placed in the nursing home. Federal reimbursement to the state for that particular individual, however, would be reduced 10%–20% from the usual reimbursement for nursing home care. This would create an incentive for the state to develop community programs.

Private patients also would be subject to the preadmission screening review. Private patients who entered despite a negative review would have a three-month waiting period before Medicaid took effect after determination of eligibility, unless it could be shown they had no alternative.

Rationale. This paper separated the nursing home cost problem from the development of a community support system. This recommendation would tackle the nursing home situation. Inappropriate placement in a nursing home is bad for the individual and costly for the taxpayer. Yet such placements occur because people either do not realize that they could remain in the community, or lack services. The intent of this recommendation is to give the states a fiscal incentive/penalty to develop community services and reduce the inappropriate placements. The preadmission review is assigned to the PSRO because it is an existing entity with experience in case evaluation, especially in institutional settings. It would have no case management responsibilities. I am assuming that too much role strain will be created in an agency that both *denies* services and *advocates* for disabled persons. Unless the

nursing home side is controlled, funds will not be available for community programs.

4. At the state level, an interdepartmental structure should be created
to prepare a state plan for long-term care. The plan would document the
steps the state was taking to coordinate departments and programs in
long-term care, would identify regional and local planning responsibilities,
and would identify leading case management agencies. The cost of the
planning process would be shared 80/20 federal/state. Federal approval of
the plan would result in increased federal sharing in selected federal/state
programs (e.g., Medicaid, vocational rehabilitation, special education,
etc.). The increased share could be a change in the federal/state ratio, a
per-capita-based sum, or a fixed amount. A maintenance of effort clause
would be required. This approach would provide a clear financial incentive to the states to improve service delivery, yet leave approval control in
the hands of the federal government.

Rationale. The state is an important actor in long-term care. It provides
some of the funds under Title XIX and Title XX. It funds some of its
own programs affecting the disabled. It licenses and regulates. It is
important that the state understand what it is doing in long-term care in
the interest of improvement.

5. At the local level, a two-fold strategy should be developed for meeting long-term-care needs. First would be a case management strategy. It
needs to be recognized that only a certain subset of individuals requires
case management. Many individuals and families handle their own affairs
very well. There is no need to overload a system by attempting to bring in
this group. It is important also to recognize that there is a difference
between a case manager within an agency with specific linking functions,
and case management as a community system of patient management. A
comprehensive case management or channeling system might be experi-
mented with, but should not be seen as a panacea. Rather, there should be
more case managers within specific agencies to serve as individual advocates, and case planners should be encouraged. Case management services would be established within the client sectors identified earlier. That
is, the school system would be responsible for case management of the
handicapped child and young adult; the vocational rehabilitation agency
would be responsible for case management of disabled adults; and the
Area Agencies on Aging directly or by subcontract would be responsible
for case management of elderly. Community mental health centers would
be responsible for the mentally ill. The public social service agency would
be responsible for case management of those who fit none of the above
categories or for those who fall through the cracks. The identification of
who is responsible for case management in each of the sectors would be

part of the state plan mentioned above and would be one requirement for increased federal financial participation. The federal government should establish also a demonstration program to fund associations of users to act as case managers/advocates for their particular population group.

Second, a wide range of discretionary, non-means-tested, non-case-managed services should be created at the local level, particularly for older people. These would include senior centers, telephone reassurance programs, nutrition sites, accessible recreation areas, respite care centers, and the like. Federal funding should be expanded to encourage the development of these prevention-type programs.

Rationale. The idea behind this recommendation is to build on existing forces and elements at the local level (see table 5.1), in other words, to exploit the positive forces in the community. This recommendation recognizes the need for case coordination and attempts to locate responsibility for that coordination. The recommendation assumes that no one agency can or should do all the case management. Increased federal financial participation would be available as an incentive for a state/locality to come up with a coordinated plan.

Case-managed services are often sought because more appropriate services do not exist. To avoid this system distortion, other components need to be created to help people before they need case-managed services.

6. Movement must take place toward a comprehensive national health service. Eyeglasses, dentures, and drugs are important items, particularly for the elderly, but are excluded under Medicare. Exclusion of the handicapped and disabled young adult and middle-aged populations from private health insurance benefits and, frequently, Medicaid benefits is a serious gap that reduces access to necessary service resources. This gap, too, needs to be closed. Expansion of specialized housing for handicapped and adults is required, as is improvement in mass transportation.

The program outlined above is not revolutionary, but rather is incremental and—I hope—realistic. In my opinion, however, it does build upon some of the strengths of existing long-term-care delivery mechanisms and offers the hope of an improvement in them. Despite the natural American antipathy toward planning, this is a very needed and necessary component if long-term-care services are to be improved. Long-term care promises to be a long-term problem. We should stay away from quick solutions that achieve nothing but publicity if we are really concerned about the people who need service. Careful planning, the judicious use of incentives and sanctions, and respect for what others are doing are at least some of the essentials of a successful strategy.

Appendix 1
Long-Term-Care Services Identified by
National Conference on Social Welfare

Potential Resources and Services in a
Continuum of Long-Term Care

Intramural

Definition: 24-hour residential services for long-term/intermittent/acute treatment.

Federal hospitals (VA, PHS)
Chronic disease hospitals
Psychiatric hospitals, county and state (adult/child)
Psychiatric hospitals (nonprofit/proprietary) (adult/child)
Training schools for developmentally disabled (e.g., blind, deaf, and mentally retarded
Special residential facilities for mentally retarded
Residential special facilities for children (e.g., crippled children)
Special facilities for aging (geriatric institutes, homes for the elderly)
Hospital extended care units
General hospital special units (e.g., burns)
General hospital medical and surgical units
General hospital psychiatric units
Skilled nursing homes
Intermediate care facilities
Personal care, shelter care, board and care homes
Congregate living; group homes

Intermediate alcohol and drug treatment units; detoxification units
State and local forensic psychiatry units
Detention centers; jail units
Halfway houses and other special facilities for alcoholics and drug abusers
Special living arrangements for the elderly (apartments, communities)
Summer camps for disabled and handicapped

Intermediate

Definition: Nonresidential, less than 24-hours; person goes to agency or service locale.

Information, screening and referral services
Crisis intervention
Hospital emergency rooms
Income maintenance and employment assistance, state and local social
    services
Neighborhood health centers
Senior citizen or geriatric centers
Individual and group practitioners (health, mental health, social services,
    physical therapy, chiropractic, other)
Health Maintenance Organizations (HMOs), outpatient diagnostic and
    treatment services
Community mental health centers
State and local social service agencies for counseling and related services
Medical, dental, physical therapy and behavioral clinics (including univer-
    sities)
State and local public health departments
Drop-in clinics
Family planning clinics
Local children's bureaus
Sheltered workshops
State and local vocational rehabilitation services
Vocational education
Employment counseling
School special education classes
Special day training schools
Adult activity centers for mentally retarded and other handicapped
Recreational-therapeutic activity programs for persons-at-risk
Day camps for disabled
Day care centers (adult/child)
Night/day partial hospitalization

Extramural

Definition: Services are provided at the site of the problem, i.e., home,
school, and all of the facilities listed under Intramural and Intermediate.
Services are provided by an individual worker or practitioner and/or
agency personnel.

Spectrum of Extramural Services
House Calls

Medical   Crisis intervention
Psychological   Screening
Social work   Diagnostic/assessment
                                 Therapies
                                 Counseling

Home health visitations (nursing)
Home-delivered meals
Nutrition counseling
Personal care services
Homemaker services
Chore services
Shopping assistance
Income assistance and management counseling
Legal services and counseling
Vocational counseling
Employment counseling
Homebound teaching
Public library homebound services
Education TV programs for specific audience
Transportation services
Special support groups: Widow-to-Widow, Reach-to-Recovery, etc.
Friendly visitor
Telephone reassurance

Appendix 2

A report by the American Public Welfare Association listed 12 categories
of services needed by long-term-care persons, as follows:
  (1) Protective and advocacy services
  (2) Comprehensive functional assessment services
  (3) Growth services comprising activities aimed at enhancing skills

(4) Independent living services
(5) 24-hour emergency services
(6) Services that support family members who may undertake to care for an impaired member
(7) Services that enable elderly or handicapped people to remain in their own homes
(8) Services that provide appropriate social care arrangements on a temporary or permanent basis for elderly or handicapped adults or children who cannot remain or be cared for by others in their own homes
(9) Services to help older persons understand and deal with changes in their interpersonal relationships and crisis situations
(10) Services that provide for participation in social activities and constructive use of free time
(11) Child welfare services
(12) Adequate health care

Notes

1. Commission on Chronic Illness, *Care of the Long-Term Patient* (Cambridge, Mass.: Harvard University Press, 1956), pp. 19–20.

2. Congressional Budget Office, "Long-Term Care for the Elderly and Disabled," February 1977, and "Long-Term Care: Actuarial Cost Estimates," August 1977; Eddie Correia, "National Health Insurance, Welfare Reform, and the Disabled: Issues in Program Reform," Office of the Assistant Secretary for Planning and Evaluation, U.S. Dept. of Health, Education and Welfare, August 1976; Tom Joe and Judy Meltzer, "Policies and Strategies for Long-Term Care," Health Policy Program, University of California, San Francisco, May 14, 1976; William Pollak, "Federal Long-Term Care Strategy: Options and Analysis," The Urban Institute, October 17, 1973, revised February 25, 1974; U.S. Department of Health, Education, and Welfare, "Program Design Choices for Long-Term-Care Legislative Initiative—Decision Memorandum," Office of the Secretary, August 1974; U.S. Department of Health, Education, and Welfare, "Long-Term-Care Services Legislative Proposal," Office of the Secretary, October 19, 1976.

3. *Major Options in Long Term Care,* University Health Policy Consortium, Brandeis University, Waltham, Mass., 1980.

4. Sue C. Hawkins and Donald E. Rigby, "Effect of SSI on Medicaid Caseloads and Expenditures," *Social Security Bulletin* 43, no. 2 (February 1979): 3–14.

5. HEW Task Force Report 1978, Tables 2 & 3.

6. *Health, U.S.A.,* 1978, p. 419.

7. Robert Solem, and Michael Garrich, "The Community-Based Care Project: Options in Long-Term Care or Support" (Paper presented at the 20th Annual Meeting, Gerontological Society, 1978).

8. Robert Agranoff, *Dimension of Service Integration,* Project Share, no. 13, April 1979.

9. Gerben DeJong, "The Movement for Independent Living: Origins, Ideology, and Implications for Disability Research," University Centers for International Rehabilitation, Michigan State University, East Lansing, Mich., March 1, 1979.

10. J. Callahan, L. Diamond, J. Giele, and R. Morris, "Responsibility for Families for Their Severely Disabled Elders," University Health Policy Consortium, Brandeis University, Waltham, Mass., July 1979.

11. Henry T. Ireys, "The Health Care Needs of Chronically Disabled Children and Their Families" (Paper presented for the Select Panel for the Promotion of Child Health, Center for the Study of Families and Children, Vanderbilt Institute for Public Policy Studies, November 5, 1979), p. 9.

12. For a discussion of the political, organizational, and personal factors involved in intersystem planning, see Jim L. Munro, "Intersystem Action Planning: Criminal and Non-Criminal Justice Agencies," *Public Administration Review* (July/August, 1976), pp. 390–97.

13. "The Future for Social Services in the United States," National Conference on Social Welfare, Columbus, Ohio, 1977.

14. "The Integration and Coordination of Social Services through a National Personal Social Service System," American Public Welfare Association, December 1978.

15. See Ireys, op. cit., for a detailed discussion of this sector of the long-term-care service system.

16. *The Future of Long Term Care in the U.S.,* National Conference on Social Welfare, February 1977. See Appendix 1 for complete list of services.

17. "Report of the Task Force on Long-Term Care," American Public Welfare Association, December 1978. See Appendix 2 for listing of services.

18. Dennis Beatrice, "A Core Service Package for Long-Term-Care Demonstration Projects," University Health Policy Consortium, Brandeis University, Waltham, Mass., July 1979. See also OARS.

19. *Long Term Care for the Elderly and Disabled,* Washington, D.C., Congressional Budget Office, February 1977.

20. HEW Task Force 1978, Table 3.

21. Ibid., Table 14.

22. Review Committee of the Social Welfare Series, *Meeting the Needs—Managing the System* (Worcester, Mass., 1973).

23. Technical Notes prepared by Eileen Wolff, Office of the Assistant Secretary for Planning and Evaluation, DHEW, May 1, 1978.

24. Sol Levine and Paul E. White, "Exchange as a Conceptual Framework for the Study of Inter-Organizational Relationships," *Administrative Science Quarterly* 5, no. 4 (March 1961); and Sol Levine, Paul E. White and Benjamin D. Paul, "Community Inter-Organizational Problems in Providing Medical Care in Social Services," AJPH 53, no. 8 (August 1963).

25. Eugene Litwak and Lydia Hylton, "Inter-Organizational Analysis: A Hypothesis on Coordinating Agencies," *Administrative Science Quarterly*.

26. Roland M. Warren, Stephen M. Rose, and Anne F. Burgunder, *The Structure of Urban Reform* (Lexington, Mass.: Lexington Books, 1974).

27. Ibid., p. 31.

28. Daniel Hainline and Michael Lindsey, "An Analysis of Aging Services Networks in Six Cities" (Paper presented at the Annual Meeting of the Gerontological Society, Dallas, Texas, November 1978).

29. Ibid., p. 23.

30. David Mechanic, "The Sociology of Organizations," in *The Administration of Mental Health Services,* ed. Saul Feldman (Springfield, Ill.: Charles C. Thomas, 1973), p. 150, pp. 138–66.

31. Robert Morris and Ilana Hirsch-Lescohier, "Service Integration: Real vs. Illusory Solutions to Welfare Dilemmas," Brandeis University, June 1977.

32. For additional information on the results of service integration, see the Project Share Series including "Managing the Human Service 'System': What Have We Learned from Service Integration?" (No. 4, August 1977) and "Dimension of Service Integration" (No. 13, April 1979).

33. Michael Aiken, et al., *Coordinating Home Services* (San Francisco: Jossey-Bass, 1975).

34. William Datel, Jane G. Murphy, and Philip L. Pollack, "Outcome in a Deinstitutionalization Program Employing Service Integration Methodology," *Journal of Operational Psychiatry* 9, no. 1 (1978): 5.

35. Department of Health, Education, and Welfare, *Community Life Association from 1970–1975,* Washington, D.C., January 1976.

36. Raymond M. Steinberg, "Case Coordination: Lessons from the Past for Future Program Models" (Paper presented at the National Conference on Social Welfare, Los Angeles, Calif., May 24, 1978).

37. For a discussion of these strategies, see David Austin, "Administrative Considerations in the Improvement of Human Services at State and Local Levels," School of Social Work, University of Texas at Austin, Tex., January 1980.

38. See Warren, op. cit., pp. 60–66, for a detailed analysis of the preventing, blunting, repelling behavior of the interorganizational field.

39. Roland L. Warren, *The Community in America* (Chicago: Rand McNally, 1963).

40. Sydney Gardner, "Policy Space: A Sharper Perspective on Local Decision Making," in *Human Services Management: Parameters for Research,* ed. Michael J. Murphy and Thomas Glynn (Washington, D.C.: International City Management Association, 1978), pp. 19–20.

41. Janet Z. Giele, "Social Policy and the Family," *American Review of Sociology* (1979), p. 282.

42. Orion White, Jr., and Bruce L. Gates, "Statistical Theory and Equity in the Delivery of Social Services," *Public Administration Review,* no. 1 (January/February 1974).

43. Ibid., p. 44.

44. Stephen J. Miller, "The Education Experience of Interns," Brandeis University, 1968.

45. Bernard Frieden, "Defining the Objectives of Human Services in Local Government," in Murphy and Glynn, p. 5.

46. Morris and Lescohier, pp. 41–42.

47. Aiken, et al., pp. 147–69. (See table 5.2)

48. James J. Callahan, Jr., *Single Agency Option for Long-Term Care,* University Health Policy Consortium, Waltham, Mass., 1979. (See table 5.3)

49. Robert Agranoff, *Dimension of Service Integration,* Project Share, No. 13, April 1979.

50. William Pollak, *Expanding Health Benefits for the Elderly* (Washington, D.C.: The Urban Institute, 1977); Callahan, op. cit.

51. Barbara Ishizaki, Leonard Gottesman, Stacey Mong MacBride, "Determinants of Model Choice for Service Management Functions," *Gerontologist* 19, no. 1 (August 1979): 388.

6

Finding the Money and
Paying for Long-Term-Care
Services
The Devil's Briarpatch

William D. Fullerton

I. Introduction

The purpose of this paper is to discuss the strengths and weaknesses of possible additional sources of financing to meet the increased costs of providing long-term-care services. The paper also discusses selected types of reimbursement schemes to pay for these services.

The terms "financing" and "reimbursement" are separated in the usual way: financing means the source of funds—whether public or private—which pay for long-term-care services; reimbursement means the terms or conditions under which these funds are paid to those providing the covered services.

The paper will not discuss organization or program administration, although there is some discussion of administrative problems in the section which addresses the issues raised by open-ended versus limited federal grants.

The paper will deal primarily with sources of funding and types of reimbursement for services—not sources of funding for creating or maintaining a work force or other delivery resources. There will be a discussion of how well the various sources of financing and reimbursement methods relate to resource creation and maintenance.

Long-term-care services are now funded through a variety of sources and that situation will no doubt continue. Realistically, as the need for long-term-care services grows with an aging population, the practical decision is not to settle on a single source of funding but rather to find the best sources of additional funding. Attempting to find the *one* best source of funds or the *one* best reimbursement system for long-term care would be useless.

It is simply not possible to consider major shifts in existing financing for the foreseeable future. That will explain what some readers may view as undue concern with practicability and political feasibility. This concern also explains why I have included a discussion of provisions to assure the maintenance of current funding levels from various sources, both public and private, as new sources are added.

II. Financing Long-Term-Care Services

The following sources of financing have been selected for discussion and evaluation:

1. Payroll financing on a prepaid basis, such as that used in the hospital insurance part of Medicare Part A.
2. Federal general revenues, including some discussion of allocation methods such as matching grants, open-ended or closed, and grants where no matching effort is required.
3. Taxes on alcohol and tobacco.
4. Value-added taxes.
5. Contributions from those who choose to join a program offering long-term-care services which are matched or subsidized through other sources of funds, such as state or federal general revenues. This type of financing is used for the supplemental health insurance part of Medicare Part B.
6. Tax deductions and tax credits acting as a stimulant to increase or maintain private spending.
7. Cost sharing.

When considering the advantages and disadvantages of these approaches, it seems best to begin by discussing the criteria that should be used to evaluate the selected sources of funding. The first part of the paper attempts to do that. An evaluation using these criteria is then made of each source of funding.

The paper applies the same test for possible reimbursement methods for long-term-care services—first by setting out the evaluation criteria and then following with the evaluation. In this part of the paper there is also some discussion of the relationships which may exist between sources of funding and methods of paying for long-term-care services.

There is a separate section on the relationship between national health insurance proposals and the set of issues usually encumbered by the term "the long-term-care problem." While not directly related to financing methods, this section is related to questions of major priorities among national needs. And besides, it satisfies the author's need to talk about a relationship he believes is not generally well understood among health and social policymakers.

A. Criteria for Evaluating Sources of Financing Long-Term Care

Any source of financing for long-term care should be evaluated on the basis of the following criteria. Listed below are the criteria and my reasons for including each.

1. *Inflationary impact.*—For the foreseeable future, concerns over inflation will greatly influence the attitude of policymakers at all levels toward sources selected for funding new programs. The attitude of the Carter administration toward funding sources of national health insurance illustrates the point clearly. For example, a payroll tax would be viewed with less favor than would raising the same amount of funds from general revenues, because the payroll tax is viewed as inflationary. An increase in general revenues—derived from corporate and personal income taxes— would be viewed as anti-inflationary.[1]

2. *Extent of income redistribution effects.*—Most of the people who will be involved in major changes in the sources of funding for long-term-care services will be concerned about the extent to which the financing choices will redistribute money from higher-income to lower-income individuals and families. The usual arguments of equity versus ability to pay cannot avoid becoming a part of the debate, even if, as has often been the case, it will not be discussed directly. Thus, the same kinds of arguments about income redistribution that arise when income tax changes are proposed will have to be faced with regard to long-term-care financing. Those who would attempt two goals in one proposal—finding a source of funds for long-term-care services and redistributing income—could accomplish neither very easily. Ideally, the source would be as neutral as possible on this score if acceptability is the primary goal.

3. *Effects of growth of program over time.*—Clearly, in fields such as long-term care, where the population at risk, and therefore the total need, is expected to grow substantially over time (with more predictability to this change than to most other economic and social factors in modern life), it can be very important to select a financing source which will more or less automatically produce increased funds as increased needs arise. Thus, an income source that had this growth characteristic would have to be given preference over one that did not.

4. *Effect of financing source on resource creation.*—Reimbursement policy no doubt has more effect on the impetus to create and maintain the resources which produce needed long-term-care services than does the source of the fund. Yet there is enough relationship between resource creation and the basic financing source that some discussion of these relationships is warranted. Those who must invest in the resources are bound to take into account, in making capital spending decisions, their perception of the reliability of the source of the income over time, and this reliability is in part a function of funding. For example, the annual appropriation process of general revenues is likely to be viewed as much more subject to change—including major cutbacks—than an earmarked tax set aside to pay for long-term-care services.

5. *Ease of administration.*—While not an overriding concern, and clearly of less importance than most other factors, the ease of administering the funds-gathering mechanism has pertinence to appraisal of a financing method. For example, a national value-added tax, while not new to most western nations, would create the need to establish a major tax-collecting mechanism not now in place. On the other hand, a surcharge on the personal or corporate income tax or alcohol and tobacco taxes might involve the least new effort, since no new tax rules or mechanisms need be established.

6. *Political acceptability.*—While it could be said with much truth that the political acceptability of any one or combination of funding sources should be at least roughly equal to the sum of the values of its advantages and disadvantages under the criteria already discussed, there is more to it than these purely objective calculations. Political acceptability of a new program and its major element—funding—depends as much on the time at which it is put forth as it does on any other factor or set of factors. The changes over time are a function of national mood, of the business cycle, and of other systematic and chance factors. The period of the mid '60s was, of course, the time when many new programs gained national ac-ceptance. For example, the programs of Medicare and federal aid to elementary and secondary education had long been proposed and dis-cussed, and both were finally enacted in 1965—and both cost huge sums even in the dollars of those days.

Political acceptability of financing mechanisms follow their own cycle. For example, the possibility of adding a payroll tax to finance long-term-care services is as remote now as financing *any* new program, no matter how politically desirable it may otherwise be, through the payroll tax mechanism. In fact, it is probably a waste of time and paper to consider that possibility.

Some may reject completely the consideration of political acceptability in this context, arguing that what should be proposed is what is right rather than what is acceptable—that to do otherwise is to subvert the policymaking process to the vagaries of the political winds. I argue that political possibilities must be taken into account in making policy if prog-ress is to be made.

B. Evaluation of Selected Financing Mechanisms

Before beginning our discussion of the possible sources of financing for long-term-care services, it will be worth reviewing briefly the possible relationships between eligibility and financing in a long-term-care pro-gram. First, of course, there need be no direct connection between financing and eligibility. Under the Medicaid program, for example, eligibility arises out of income and medical status, and no regular contribution by the patient is permitted.

Medicare is just the opposite. Contributions made during working years make beneficiaries eligible for hospital insurance (Part A) when the worker and his dependents turn 65.[2] Payment of a monthly premium permits a beneficiary to be eligible for supplementary medical insurance (Part B).

Some proposals for health benefits—such as Senator Russell B. Long's (D., La.) proposal for catastrophic health insurance, introduced in March 1971—require contributions from individuals but do not tie eligibility to the contributions. Under that plan virtually every American is eligible, but only those with wage or self-employment income would pay the special payroll tax designed to support the program. Many people who would be eligible would make no contribution. The simple conclusion seems to be first, that if there is no earmarked tax or individual contribution to finance the program, there can be no tie between eligibility and contributions, and second, that even if there is an individual tax or contribution, eligibility need not be related to it. Those who believe strongly in social insurance as the way to deal with serious risks shared by virtually all the population comprise the source of support for that approach in long-term care, including tying contributions either directly, or through employment, to eligibility. While social insurance proponents are by no means unanimous in their view on financing long-term care through social insurance, existing support for social insurance financing of such care is based on the argument that people will perceive the program in a much more favorable and responsible light if those who receive the benefits are construed as having paid for them (in whole or in part) in an insurance sense. It is simply the classical case for financing the social security program in the way it is funded.

1. *Payroll taxes.*—Discussion of this tax as a source to finance long-term-care services can be mercifully quick. *There is no significant chance that an increase in payroll taxes will be enacted by any Congress over the next several years for this or any other purpose.* Indeed, it is quite possible that scheduled increases in payroll taxes will be postposed or eliminated altogether.

There is, therefore, no need to discuss the progressivity (or lack of it), ease of administration, or any other criterion with respect to this sort of tax.

2. *Federal general revenues—variation 1—open-end formula matching to states or localities.*—The model for this approach is the Aid to Families with Dependent Children (AFDC) or Medicaid programs. The federal

government uses general revenues to match expenditures made by the states under a formula designed to assist lower per capita income states at more generous rates than higher per capita income states.

How does this method fare when the evaluation criteria are applied? Open-ended federal matching would not get high marks on inflationary impact. Use of this financing method by the Medicaid program has generated large increases in federal expenditures, with no substantial increases in benefits or liberalization of eligibility standards. In large part, of course, Medicaid expenditures rose rapidly because the health costs it paid for were rising very rapidly. In the period 1966–72, the numbers of people on public assistance rolls (and, therefore, automatically eligible for Medicaid) increased dramatically. The point that will (or should) be made is that this method did nothing to prevent or slow down inflation in health care. Perhaps it even stimulated increased costs.

Because the source of funds is federal general revenues matched usually with state general revenues, income redistribution effects derive from the tax structure which raises the funds. In general, federal funds are raised in a more progressive fashion than state funds because states rely heavily on real estate and sales taxes, which are regressive.

It is important to note that the federal funding mechanism for Medicaid has meant that federal monies were more or less automatically appropriated to meet increased expenditures. There were three major reasons that accounted for increased expenditures: more eligible people, improvements in the benefit structure, and inflation in health care costs.

Of course, the rapid increases in Medicaid costs created problems at both federal and state levels. However, the primary reaction of the federal government (after some limits on eligibility were put in early in the program in 1967) has been not to limit eligibility or reduce benefits. Instead, HHS has sought to change the program in ways designed to restrain cost increases through improved administration, reimbursement limits, and increased efforts to curb fraud and abuse.

Perhaps the most favorable aspect of this method of financing is its flexibility. By using virtually automatic appropriations, funding can increase to accommodate persons newly eligible for benefits, to expand benefits, and to cover inflation in the costs of the covered benefits. It also retains, over time, the same ratio of federal to state and local funds without the need to readjust the appropriations level every year in Congress. This method does respond well to needs for resource creation. The great increase in nursing home beds over the last two decades was clearly in response to programs (beginning with the 1960 Kerr-Mills program) which financed care using open-ended federal matching funds for state expenditures.

Clearly this source of funding gets high marks on ease of administration because the tax collection systems at both federal and state levels are already in place.

On the political side, this method gets some bad marks for features already described as strengths under other criteria. Its ability to respond easily to increases in program costs subjects it to attack as not being efficient or controllable according to today's political rhetoric. Moreover, the Medicaid experience, even if not completely comparable, will be used to attack cost estimates of proposed new programs and hopefully thus to restrict or defeat altogether proposed legislation. Nonetheless, of the existing sources, only the restricted grant approach gets higher political marks because the other sources of public funds are subject to even more severe attacks.

3. *Federal general revenues—variation 2—restricted grants to states and localities.*—Under a limited grant the appropriations committee can appropriate less than but no more than the dollar limit set out in the basic authorizing statute. For example, Title V of the Social Security Act (Maternal and Child Health and Crippled Children's Services) authorizes expenditures of \$399,864,200. In fiscal year 1980, the Congress actually appropriated \$345,000,000. In a program like Medicaid, which offers to match whatever the states spend under their programs, there is neither a total dollar limit in the authorizing legislation *nor any effective way the congressional appropriating process can set a total dollar limit.* The Congress has year after year passed supplemental appropriations to meet unexpected Medicaid expenditures. It has essentially no choice but to put up its share of total state Medicaid expenditures. This method of direct public financing gets the highest marks of any existing source of funds in overall political feasibility. First, the funding source tends to be progressive in nature. Second, the implications of the restricted grant approach —that the amount of funds is limited and appropriated each year— matches current tight-spending attitudes because it does not escape in any way from the detailed scrutiny of the federal budgeting and appropriation process. Title XX of the Social Security Act (Grants to States for Services) is a prime example of a preference for restricted grants over open-ended grants. Part A of Title IV of the Social Security Act created an open-ended cash public assistance program providing social services as well as cash grants to poor families with dependent children. In the early 1970s the social service expenditure part of the program was rising so fast that Congress decided to cap the program. Thus, Title XX was created and it became one of the largest limited-grant type programs.

The restricted grant is also a form of budgeting. It represents the amount Congress decided to spend on the set of activities covered by the grant. The question of budgeting mechanisms—how much each state gets— raises administrative considerations beyond the scope of this paper.

The limited grant, however, must be given low marks according to other criteria. This approach is more difficult to adjust to growing needs over time. It is not dependable or stable, in the sense that it is subject to ups and downs related to factors other than the needs of the program. Such factors as swings in the general economy, changing attitudes on federal spending (and borrowing), and even the personal vagaries of individual committee or subcommittee chairmen or other influential federal policymakers can lead to variability and instability.

Many people have in mind another consideration when comparing open-ended to restricted-grant mechanisms. To many, an open-ended grant from the federal government matched by the states will mean fairly detailed federal rules on the states concerning the purposes, coverage, and other features of the program while a restricted grant implies a minimum of federal rules. The distinction is made, however, not because it automatically follows if one is open and the other limited but because of the general conclusion that an open-ended system needs rules to contain growth in costs, while a closed end does not, the cap itself acting as the control mechanism. For example, under Medicaid, the Congress, in some cases at the request of the executive branch, has imposed additional requirements on state Medicaid plans. The original law contained 22 plan requirements, current law contains 40, and almost all require activities designed to control utilization and costs under the program. There have been many spirited debates over just how much and what kind of federal rules should be imposed in both types of systems, but discussion of these issues beyond making this one point is outside the scope of this paper.

4. *A tobacco and alcohol surcharge tax.*—There has been a continuing interest on the part of many people interested in health policy in increasing taxes paid on alcohol and tobacco and then earmarking the new funds for some specific purpose related to health. This proposal is made by some on grounds of equity, particularly when it has been put forward as part of a national health insurance plan. The idea is that people who choose to consume these products tend to use more health care than those who do not and therefore should be made to pay more than those who do not. Proponents of this idea argue that it is simply unfair to have people who choose not to use these products subsidize those who do. Of course, this unfair situation exists today and few complain about it because so much of health care costs (particularly costs of acute care) is spread over various insured populations.

Others argue that these additional taxes should be imposed to act as a disincentive to the use of such products, contending that the revenue raised from this "less-than-good" source should be used to support a "good" program like preventive health services for children. An obvious flaw in this line of reasoning is that if the "good" purpose comes to depend on the "bad" funds, funding levels may not be adequate unless use of the bad product increases. Also, of course, there is little evidence so far that increasing the price of these products will significantly lower their use.

The question then of whether a surcharge tax on alcohol and tobacco should be used to support provision of long-term-care services depends in part on how strongly people feel about the relationship between these products and health.

But perhaps most important in a pragmatic world is the question of how much of a political problem for enactment of a long-term-care program would be created by proposing such a financing source. I suggest that the amount of political antagonism which would be generated far exceeds the benefits from using this source—even though substantial amounts of funds are at stake. (For example, each penny of additional tax on a pack of cigarettes raises more than $300 million a year.) The alcohol and tobacco lobby is simply too formidable an opponent to be added to those who would already oppose any substantial increase in spending for long-term-care services. This form of tax is, of course, quite easy to administer since the tax collection mechanisms are already in place—a simple surcharge added to present computed taxes would impose only a very small burden. The impact of such a surcharge would be inflationary.

5. *A value-added tax.*—A value-added tax is one that imposes a tax on a product at each stage of manufacture related to the value added to the product during that stage. It is somewhat similar to a sales tax and shares regressiveness as a drawback. Because the tax is collected before the point of sale, however, the purchaser is not aware of the amount of the tax.

The tax increases the price of the final product and thus contributes to inflation.

Several European countries have used this form of taxation for many years, and it appears to have general acceptance. The United Kingdom is now considering more such taxes, but primarily in combination with reductions in income taxes, with no net increase in revenue.

Propositions of a value-added tax for any purpose will require establishing a new collection mechanism. Such a tax is not easy to administer because questions of just what value was added at each stage of manufacture can raise thorny accounting and related issues. Moreover, any final enactment is very likely to include exceptions and special rules necessary to placate powerful interest groups. Such provisions could substantially complicate the collection system.

Because collection totals from a value-added tax are likely to follow the business cycle, variation in the sums collected can be expected to have little or no relation to the funding needs of a long-term-care program.

In this country, principal tax policymakers only recently have proposed such a tax.[3] And while there will be strong opposition and early enactment is clearly not likely, when and if it does come, a value-added tax will, as contemplated, in the U.S., be coupled directly with other tax reductions—probably in Social Security and income tax provisions.

It would seem then that not much reliance can be put on a value-added tax as a significant new source of funds for long-term-care services.

6. *Prepaid contributions from eligibles.*—Proposals have been put forth in the Congress during the last five years which would create, as one source of income to pay for the long-term-care services, premiums from people who voluntarily enroll in a program providing entitlement to a defined set of such services. While this source was only one relatively minor source of the funding under these proposals, it would be easy to increase this source substantially. The major advantage of this method is that it does contain a strong element of prepaid insurance because payments tend to be made before need arises. These proposals would make coverage available when people become eligible for Medicare at age 65. Because the need for long-term-care services increases substantially about a decade or so later on the average, such a program has the advantage of getting support in large part from people who do not yet, but probably will at some time, need the covered services. In other words, it would be largely a prepayment system. The great advantage is clear: no new taxes would need to be imposed.

Perhaps the most serious disadvantage is that this source can be used only with an entitlement program, an approach which many people regard as highly flawed. An entitlement system under which individuals have a legal right to payment for benefits used if they qualify for such benefits, the argument goes, cannot be managed in a way to control costs effectively. While the "need" for long-term-care services cannot be effectively questioned (even to the degree acute-care services can be questioned), the idea that people are entitled to the benefits leads to utilization pressures which cannot be resisted. Moreover, those who want to see existing private sources maintained (including the assistance of the family) fear that an entitlement program will substitute public for private funds and purchased services for those now provided by family and friends. What needs further exploration is whether the premium source can be set so that there is a net increase in private spending rather than a decrease, while retaining the element of prepayment which avoids concentration of private spending at the time of need.

This source of funding is not inflationary (it may even be somewhat deflationary, particularly in the early years, because the money comes from funds otherwise available for spending and is held for a time before it is spent for long-term-care services).

The contributions are readily collected under this system because it could be added to the present system of collecting Medicare Part B premiums.

Those who cannot afford the premiums could be helped under public assistance, just as Medicaid now pays the Part B premium on behalf of those eligible for it.

7. *Tax deductions and tax credits.*—Tax deductions already may be taken for expenditures on long-term-care services. The "national health insurance system" as operated under our present tax system has some generally unappreciated quirks and idiosyncracies. Some attention has been brought to these tax provisions, such as their providing more benefits to the rich than to the poor by decreasing tax liabilities at an increased rate as income goes up (a charge which can be made about most tax deductions as compared with tax credit provisions in the Internal Revenue Code). Just about all forms of expenditures for long-term-care services can now be taken as a deduction under the tax laws.

Several questions can be explored under this general subject. First, do the existing tax provisions encourage private spending for long-term-care services, or are they merely ways to reduce the taxes of those who must pay these costs in any event? While I am aware of no specific studies to elucidate the question, I suggest that most of the spending would have occurred with or without the tax provisions. There are two exceptions. One, families with substantial incomes may find that putting an elderly family member on Medicaid can be avoided if the health-care expenditures on the elderly themselves can offset taxes based on tax rates of 50 percent to 70 percent of family income which would otherwise be payable to federal and state governments. (These lost revenues could just as well be regarded as public rather than private expenditures.) Two, the tax deductibility of long-term-care expenditures can delay to some degree the point at which people become eligible for Medicaid. Particularly in the case of institutionalization in a long-term nursing home, it is almost inevitable that an individual (or couple) will exhaust their resources in a relatively short time when nursing home costs of many hundreds of dollars must be met every month. The saving in income from deducting these costs for income tax purposes can delay the inevitable, but only for a little while.

Tax deductions and tax credits are common in the present system, of course, so additional ones should not be very burdensome on existing tax-collecting mechanisms (although there must be a point where the sheer numbers of such provisions would seriously impede the tax collection functions).

Tax credits and deductions, to the extent they result in spending which would not otherwise occur, have inflationary effects though the effects are not so large that they would be rejected on these grounds alone.

Tax credits and deductions are probably more politically acceptable than direct general revenue spending but more taxpayers are sophisticated enough today to see that forgone tax revenues have as much effect on balancing the budget as direct expenditures.

8. *Cost-sharing.*—While contributions (or premiums) and direct private spending might be considered a form of private cost-sharing of the total costs of long-term-care services, cost-sharing will be discussed in this section in its more usual meaning under insurance-type programs. Medicare has cost-sharing in both its parts, and even Medicaid can have certain limited cost-sharing features if states choose to impose them.[4]

Any substantial cost-sharing requires a mechanism—a means test—for defining those who cannot pay the cost-sharing imposed. This implies a heavy administrative effort if it were done separately for a long-term-care program, or even if an existing means-testing mechanism were to be used and cost-sharing were among the multiple benefits which had to be coordinated. Medicaid's use of means-tested programs to determine eligibility has led to a set of eligibility requirements which are simply impossible to administer without large eligibility error being introduced into the system.

Cost-sharing must also be evaluated in a long-term-care program (just as in other programs) according to its effectiveness in keeping program costs down both from its direct impact on program prices and from direct impact on utilization of covered services. The issues in this area have been the subject of many studies and meetings and are simply not within the scope of this paper.

III. Reimbursement Methods
A. Criteria for Evaluating Methods of Reimbursement for Long-Term-Care Services

1. *Definition of covered services.*—While it might not appear so at first, perhaps the most important prerequisite for operating an effective reimbursement method is as precise a definition as possible of the items or services which are to be paid for. If the definition is not precise, the program will tend to pay for services not intended to be covered. To take a simple example, suppose that a long-term-care program covered day-

care services. If the term were not defined further, care in a substandard facility (or even in a neighbor's home) might be paid for.

For the purposes of discussing all the methods of reimbursement, then, we shall presume that a precise definition of the covered items or services is required by all.

2. *Effect on resources creation.*—Clearly one of the objectives to which a reimbursement system should be directed is the creation or maintenance of an adequate number, and appropriate location, of the individuals and organizations which furnish the covered items or services.

While the primary factor determining program support for appropriate resources is the set of benefits to be covered and, as described earlier, a stable source of program funding plays a role in this support, clearly the reimbursement method selected can nullify the effect of coverage and financing. For example, if the method does not recognize the need to invest and maintain capital necessary to produce the item or services, the whole program may prove to be unsuccessful. The Medicare reimbursement formula recognizes capital needs in its coverage of interest and depreciation on capital investments.

3. *Acceptability to providers.*—This point goes beyond the one just discussed. Even if adequate allowance is made for necessary capital funds, other aspects of a reimbursement method may be, or may be perceived to be, so unfair that providers of the service may refuse to participate in the program. Even those participating may give the program a poor image if continuous and bitter bickering over reimbursement occurs.

Of course, there may be just as much process here as substance. If a reimbursement method is arrived at through or allows for negotiation and consultation with the provider community, acceptance is much more likely than in the absence of such a process, at any given level of total reimbursement.

4. *Ease of administration.*—This element speaks for itself. A method which is too complex for either the payer or the payee needs to be rejected outright. What is really involved here is to strike an acceptable balance between the need for simplicity and ease of administration on the one hand and the need for special provisions designed to assure equity or acceptability by the providers on the other.

5. *Cost effectiveness.*—Perhaps one of the most important criteria which will be used by those who make the final decisions on a reimbursement method or methods for long-term care is how cost effective the reimbursement is likely to be. It will be in this criterion that such features as

capitation, prospective payment, and reimbursement based on budgeting will get higher marks—all of them contain some element of advance limitation on expenditures. Common wisdom now attributes inflation-creating characteristics to reimbursement systems which tend to reflect costs, whether described as reasonable or total, incurred by providers. The hospital reimbursement system used under Medicare and many Blue Cross plans are subject to such criticism.

6. *Predictability of costs maximized.*—While closely related to the previous proposed criterion, this idea is somewhat different. It grows out of the experience of those who must deal with estimators—actuarial and others. If they believe that a program has a broad range of possibilities for reimbursement, or even coverage of people and services, the cost estimates will be set at the level of the combination of features which yields the highest cost.

While the estimators' vantage point is ethical and has a lot of common sense, this attitude sometimes leads to frenzied expressions of disbelief and outrage about the estimates from those who are sponsoring the plan. It is important, therefore, that the reimbursement method as part of the total plan be as predictable as possible. Only if this is done will the estimators and the sponsors be reasonably in accord on the costs of the program.

B. Evaluation of Methods of Reimbursement for Long-Term-Care Services

1. *Fee for service.*—The literature is replete with discussion of the advantages and disadvantages of reimbursement for health services on a fee-for-service basis. In essence, some argue that it is the fee-for-service system that yields high costs due to high utilization because providers determine utilization and income is increased by maximizing the number of services provided.[5]

Others argue that reimbursement on a fee-for-service basis, unlike capitation arrangements, assures that needed services will not be withheld in order to come under a capitation or other limit. These arguments have arisen in connection with private and public programs which cover acute health care services. As we begin to consider those health and social services which would make up an array of services described as long-term-care services, the considerations become somewhat different. In the first place, the major independent private practice health professionals—physicians or dentists—will continue to be paid on a fee-for-service basis for the foreseeable future. A long-term-care program of any sort will not change that. Nor would a national health insurance program of any sort remove fee for service as a method of payment.

Many (perhaps most) of those who support one or another national health insurance proposal will attempt to control the fee-for-service element in a variety of ways—budgeting, negotiated fee schedules, controls over the listing of services (the procedure terminology code), and the relative value of services.

While such controls would also prove useful in a long-term-care program for those practitioners who historically have been paid on a fee-for-service basis, a concern of specific pertinence to long-term-care legislation would be to avoid increasing the number of practitioners reimbursed on that basis. For example, psychologists, speech pathologists, physical and occupational therapists, social workers, and many other allied health professionals who would be heavily involved in a long-term-care program are now paid to some degree on such a basis, but many others are salaried or have some other financial arrangements with organized delivery systems such as hospitals, nursing homes, home health agencies, neighborhood health centers, community mental health centers, health maintenance organizations, multispecialty physician clinics, and so on.

It seems clear that any long-term-care program should avoid increasing the number of independent allied health practitioners because changing to fee-for-service arrangements would be cost-inducing and may reduce the quality of care by reducing the extent of institutional surveillance of the service. By not recognizing any other system, the program would deliberately encourage the provision of covered services in an organized setting where there are few incentives for more utilization. The actuaries ascribe higher costs—on grounds of both higher utilization and higher unit prices—to provisions which cover independent practitioners on a fee-for-service basis rather than on primarily salary arrangements.

In summary, the principal concern about fee-for-service reimbursement in a long-term-care program is that increasing the incentives for practitioners to practice on this basis will produce costs that will be higher than necessary.

Reimbursement for a long-term-care program is a function of the program's features rather than the method itself. For example, the definitions of the benefits covered determine whether a service is paid for at all. Furthermore, the payment method depends in part on what providers are reimbursed. For example, if the services of a psychiatric social worker are covered only when provided by a community mental health center or a specialized hospital, the reimbursement method that is adopted is suited to payment to an organization, not to an individual social worker.

If a long-term-care program covered all services only through such organizations, the policymakers could concentrate their efforts on the most effective method for paying organizations, and the fee-for-service model, which is needed least when relatively few covered services are provided by an individual, could be largely ignored.

2. *Capitation payments.*—The capitation method,[6] similar to that used to pay health maintenance organizations for services they provide, requires some sort of organization to receive the payments and in turn take responsibility to assure that required services are provided, either directly or through arrangements with others. Implied, too, is that a population has enrolled, or has been assigned in some other way, with the organization. This in turn suggests that the population has, in some manner or another, been made eligible to receive a set of defined benefits. The choice of this method of reimbursement then can be used only in a program which pays for defined benefits for a defined population. Consideration of the advantages of this method will be discussed on the assumption that it would be used in that sort of program.

The capitation payment method is not new to the health field, of course, and the literature is replete with discussions of actual experience and analyses of the subject. These discussions usually take the form of comparison with the fee-for-service method. To sum up many thousands of pages in one sentence, fee for service is castigated for its lack of incentives to withhold services not needed; capitation is praised for its incentives to limit services (and thus restrain costs) to those clearly needed and castigated for its incentives to withhold needed services. Further elaboration of these experiences and analyses will not be given here, but discussions of special problems in using this method for long-term-care services are clearly warranted.

While not used in long-term care, capitation has been used extensively in acute and preventive care but not nearly as much as many policymakers would like. Note the HHS efforts to stimulate growth of HMOs. Could these differences in the benefits covered lead to different results—everything else being the same—from those that could be expected to be seen in the acute-care setting? There may well be such differences. Long-term care by definition continues for an extended period once care for the individual involved begins. For some there may be no possibility of prevention or cure or alternative settings. These factors indicate that capitation for such care is clearly an area where additional analyses and, probably more importantly, experiment and demonstrations are required.

A severe difficulty for long-term care will be to define the set of benefits precisely enough to avoid disagreement between the organization making capitation payment and the organization receiving payment for services over what is to be furnished to the eligible population. The second major difficulty (at least as severe as the first) will be to get agreement on the criteria used to decide which services or set of services are needed in individual cases and on the monitoring system set up to assure compliance with these criteria. These two problems are not limited to this method of reimbursement, but a workable solution is more important under this method. Withholding services would be much easier under a set of long-term-care services than under acute-care services because the need is not so apparent and general agreement on questions of necessity is almost totallly absent. (The prepaid health plan experiences in California could very easily be repeated in a long-term-care program if these and other concerns are not carefully handled.) What may be needed to meet this problem are special monitoring and ombudsman activities not now fully developed anywhere.

The necessity for these monitoring devices suggests that the capitation method may not be as easy to administer as it appears. Moreover, while retrospective, reasonable cost reimbursement is now in high disfavor. Retrospective payment was, nonetheless, regarded as clearly superior compared with paying on the basis of billed charges when Medicare was enacted. Some activity in measuring costs and retrospective review of what has happened will also be necessary under the capitation method. The administering agency will need information and a clear set of policies to guide the process of arriving at the capitation rate.

The Medicare program can relate its capitation payment rate to the rate used by a health maintenance organization for non-Medicare enrollees, because health maintenance organizations enroll large populations for benefits similar to those covered under Medicare. This is not true in the case of long-term-care services because there are no health maintenance organizations which cover long-term-care services.

Thus, the administering agency, public or private, will need sufficient information on the costs and their reasonableness to assure that the capitation rate is not excessive. Decisions will need to be made about whether to have a retroactive element in the system in order to avoid windfall benefits to the organization or whether a system for modifying future capitation rates should reflect retrospective views of actual experience.

With today's emphasis on introducing competitive elements into the health care financing system, it is important to explore such possibilities in the reimbursement system for long-term care. There are several possible methods for setting the capitation rate.

For example, bids could be requested from long-term-care service delivery organizations, and the lowest bid meeting with specifications accepted. This is clearly theoretical, since there are virtually no such organizations in existence now. And even if more than one bid were received, the loser could hardly expect to get a contract from someone else and would immediately go out of business.

While this "pure" form of competition would not be possible, there may be other methods which could be considered to introduce elements of competition into the system.

For example, a negotiation system, under which representatives of major purchasers of health care services (those who pay taxes or contribute out-of-pocket to finance the program) sit on one side of the table and representatives of the providers sit on the other, should be carefully considered for its advantages.

Also, the organization which receives the capitation payment could be required to arrange for some of the covered services to be provided on a competitive basis. For example, a locally based delivery system could take bids on the provision of nursing home care and use a number of low bidders or pay those willing to supply the service at the low-bid rate with priority given to purchase from the low bidders, particularly when the total acute-care bed supply in the area is more than adequate.

3. *Vouchering.*—The notion that people can be given vouchers with which to purchase certain long-term-care services implies that there is some set of entitlement criteria which must be met by individuals before they can receive the vouchers. Theoretically, entitlement could be universal or limited to those in need as defined under a means test. However, several difficult decisions would have to be made. The first question would be how to decide which criteria would govern the amount and perhaps type of the voucher. In other words, some sort of need test would have to be established, not for determining economic means, but for determining the need for specific services.

Second, it is difficult to see how adequate control over the cost and quality of the services covered can be put into effect if, as a voucher system assumes, the transactions are between individuals and providers.

Third, a mechanism for assisting those who cannot be expected to make rational purchasing decisions for themselves—those found to be legally incompetent, as well as others—will be needed.

I suggest that, once these three points are adequately addressed, the "vouchering" system would not look like one any longer. Outside agencies would have made decisions about the extent of need for the services and who could use the vouchers and how someone else could use them on behalf of the incompetent. Necessary controls over cost and quality would also be set (which, no doubt, would have to be imposed eventually if not initially), and these would largely govern individual-to-provider transactions.

IV. Long-Term Care and National Health Insurance:
The Reluctant Disconnection

The relationship between the development and consideration of various national health insurance proposals and the need for long-term-care services has been frustrating to many people concerned about long-term-care issues.

National health insurance issues, strategies, and tactics have been a more important force in health policy generally than is usually appreciated. Issues such as reimbursement, health facilities planning, programs for the poor, and so on have all been affected to some degree or other (some adversely) by considerations of broader national health insurance goals by various public and private groups.

In long-term-care circles, national health insurance has been an especially strong force, sometimes in the direction of focusing attention on long-term-care issues and at other times seeming to ignore those issues or to put them aside for the time being.[7]

Even those forces in the national health insurance arena which have urged the most far-reaching changes in health care delivery and financing have balked at dealing with long-term-care issues (except for the usual study and demonstration provision).

Why is this so? I suggest that the answer goes something like this.

"Yes, we health policymakers know that long-term care is a large and largely unresolved set of issues. Yes, we know the demographics—that the problem will get much worse and something needs to be done.

"But, we are not sure what to do; the potential costs are so large as to be mind-boggling even for those who never talk in terms of less than a hundred million dollars. And anyway, there are other, more pressing, problems we do know how to handle and at a more reasonable cost."

In sum, I would suggest that key policymakers, in and out of Congress, have realized that long-term care is a problem and that it will have to be resolved someday—but they have decided that the time for resolution is not now. The attitude persists.

V. General Conclusions

My four major conclusions on financing long-term care are based, in part at least, on the analysis and discussion in the earlier parts of this paper.

A. *Existing sources of public funds for long-term-care services can at best be maintained at current levels—with little future increase.*

In the foreseeable future, given the increasing proportions of non-producers to producers in this country, primarily as a result of the aging of the population, it will not be politically feasible to increase substantially the amount of funds from traditional sources such as general revenues and payroll taxes for financing social welfare programs. The public and private statements of key policymakers in Congress and the executive branch have recognized and supported this conclusion.

B. *Because substantial increases in traditional sources of public spending cannot be relied upon, the government should encourage increased private spending and should find new forms of public financing acceptable for the purposes of funding long-term-care services.*

Previous discussions by policymakers generally on the political tactics necessary to get more of the same general revenues or payroll tax (or other special excise taxes) spent on long-term care have encountered dead ends—and will not produce results given the political situation in the country. Too little discussion and thought have been given to devising new ways to stimulate private spending, new forms of public financing, and other ideas which will have greater long-run potential for acceptance. The need to deal with the emerging long-term-care problem is generally recognized by key policymakers. What we need now are new ideas that they can explore for dealing with the problem.

C. *In both financing of and reimbursement for long-term-care services, housing for the aged has important consequences which simply cannot be ignored.*

This paper would be incomplete without at least some attention paid to housing for the aged. When older people congregate in their living arrangements, the delivery of services becomes more efficient. A service worker visitng people in their own homes can obviously provide many more occasions (units) of service in a given period if there is little time or expense between visits. Second, informal helping arrangements are much more likely to develop in congregate housing with a resulting decrease in the need for services from outside parties or organizations. Third, provision of a meal or meals for a group of people is not only more efficient, it also permits socialization, which is important to older people and thereby reduces the demand for services which arises among populations of aged who are isolated from society generally.

Fourth, the quick availability of primary health care services—such as those that might be provided by a physician's assistant or nurse practitioner—which congregate living makes possible, is more efficient and also contributes to the overall quality of care.

While all these reasons have validity, I do *not* mean that they should be the major reason for the creation of such housing. Studies show that some older people like such living arrangements and others do not. None should be forced into unacceptable arrangements solely for the sake of some cold measure of efficiency. Yet the advantages outlined above can be applied to the individual as well as the program and in my judgment are too often not fully considered when making public housing policy decisions.

D. *Expenditures for long-term-care services, no matter how precisely defined or effectively reimbursed, are likely to get out of control unless total expenditures are limited in some fashion.*

Given the inflation rate in the health industry, primarily arising from increases in the amount of services provided and our inability—so far at least—to control that inflation, the situation in long-term care will be even worse. The need for long-term-care benefits is much more subjective, and its nature less definable, than that for acute care services. No widespread, effective reimbursement systems or utilization review systems have been established, even for nursing home services, and, as the Kutza paper states so well, there is no agreement whatsoever on what is "needed" or "wanted" by the public in long-term care, even if agreement on the set of services covered were easily reached.

I believe that it is possible to design systems that meet these problems and to stimulate new ideas in these areas.

In order to lift the spirits somewhat of those readers who have concluded by now that we are dealing with a virtually hopeless situation, I have developed a proposal for discussion which may solve in many ways the dilemmas already discussed. I believe others can also be developed. The proposal is set out in enough detail to permit fairly specific discussion but is hardly a proposal refined to the point of drafting as a bill in Congress. It is my hope and intent that the proposal is both new enough and controversial enough to stir additional thought and attention to the serious issues before us.

VI. A Proposal for Financing Long-Term Care
A. Proposal

1. Permit federal taxpayers, beginning with the taxable year in which age 40 is reached to deposit 2 percent of taxable income (no less) up to a maximum of $1,000 a year (including Social Security benefits as income on which deposits may be based) into a special individual private "long-term-care" account established with a bank, insurance company, investment firm, or similar agent. The first $250 in deposits would count as a tax credit and the balance as a tax deduction. The private accounts in which the funds are deposited would be required to meet the same kind of federal requirements which currently apply to Keough and individual retirement accounts. Earnings on the invested deposits would accrue to the

individual's account and would not be taxable. Individuals filing joint returns could split total income between them for tax purposes.

Expenditures from an individual's special long-term-care account could not be made until the individual reached age 65, and then could be made only to purchase either actual services from a federally defined set of long-term-care services or federally certified private insurance policies covering nursing home services from the defined set. In the event funds from the account are used to buy insurance covering nursing home care, payments could not exceed 10 percent of the account in any one year. Certified private policies insuring nursing home care would backed by a reinsurance system funded by the federal government for nursing home expenditures in excess of $50,000 for any one individual. Payment to nursing homes whether directly from long-term-care accounts or from insurance policies, would be set through negotiations among nursing home associations, insurers, and the federal and state governments. However, in administering private health insurance for nursing home care, two aspects are vitally important to keep the benefit from being abused. First, an effective system (backed up by fiscal incentives if possible) for determining when the care is needed must be developed and found acceptable by all parties—patients, nursing homes, insurers, and government. Second, government would need to play an important role in the negotiations which establish nursing home reimbursement rates.

Funds once deposited in long-term-care accounts could not be withdrawn, except for the specified purposes. Any balance in the funds at death, before or after age 65, could be willed to a surviving spouse's account or could be added to the estate, with 75 percent counted for purposes of federal estate taxes. Long-term-care services would have to be paid for out of the fund rather than from other monies of the individual.

2. Amend the Medicaid program to mandate the same federally defined set of long-term-care services to (1) all Medicaid eligibles age 75 and older, and (2) all SSI recipients eligible on the basis of disability.

3. Establish a national lottery which would be set at a level designed to raise $2 billion in the first full year of operation with gradually increasing amounts thereafter. Half of the proceeds of the lottery would be used to finance the benefits mandated above (both federal and state shares).

4. Allocate the remaining half of the proceeds from the national lottery to the states on a basis related to aged population for creating resources to deliver the defined set of benefits, establishing and operating channeling agencies, and making long-term-care services available to those who need them but are not eligible under the provisions set out above.

5. Modify the Social Security benefit structure so that beginning at age 75 the benefits will increase 5 percent.

B. Discussion

Section 1.—This part of the proposal is designed to increase substantially private funds available to individuals during the years when the risk of requiring long-term-care services is greatest. The purpose is to establish a program for accumulating funds over a person's working life which will be available later. In this sense it is like the Social Security program. But rather than pooling the funds publicly, they are kept in private individual accounts, and in this sense the proposal more closely resembles the Keough plan for the self-employed or the individual retirement account, under which individuals are encouraged to save for their old age.

The tax credit–tax deduction provision is designed to encourage participation by lower- and middle-income taxpayers as well as higher-income taxpayers. (For the lower-income population a tax credit permits deposit in the special account without changes in current net disposable income.)

There could be significant cost to the federal government in this part of the proposal in the form of tax expenditures, but because of the tax deduction feature and substantial interest earnings over time, many more total dollars would be available for spending on long-term-care services than the tax expenditures. Moreover, tax expenditure funding is politically the least troublesome way to spend federal funds today. In addition, the creation of substantial amounts of private funds which can be used by savings institutions, insurers, and others as investment capital would be a substantial political asset for the proposal. In the current economic climate the insurance and banking industry might find the proposal quite intriguing.

The provision permitting a limited amount of the funds in the long-term-care accounts to be used to purchase insurance against the costs of nursing home care is made essentially to permit and encourage private insurance to move into this field (with substantial government involvement). Nursing home care, among all those in any set of long-term-care services will always be the most expensive and the least affordable, even if an individual who needs the care has reached age 65 with substantial amounts invested in a long-term-care fund. It is, therefore, more susceptible to the application of insurance than other long-term-care services.

The proposal would permit an individual to will the special long-term-care account to a surviving spouse without being subject to any estate tax, provided, of course, that expenditures from the spouse's fund were limited to long-term-care expenditures. If the account were not willed to a surviving spouse in that fashion, 75 percent rather than the full amount, would be counted as an asset of the estate for federal estate tax purposes. This provision furnishes another incentive for the creation and maintenance of the special account, and, more importantly, avoids incentives for spending all the funds before death. (Relatives would have a stake in seeing that not all of the funds were spent.)

Setting the eligible age at 40 is arbitrary, but at about that age people begin to see their parents facing long-term-care problems and thoughts of their own status in old age may come more often. Moreover, obligations for educating children are over or their end is in sight.

The 2 percent figure is arbitrary, also, and could be set at a higher or lower amount after some actuarial calculations are made.

Section 2.—Despite the availability of the program described under 1, there will be poor people of all ages who need long-term-care services but cannot afford them. Thus, this part of the proposal would require that state Medicaid plans cover the same set of defined long-term-care services paid for from individual long-term-care accounts. Because it will take years before the individual accounts of substantial numbers of the aged are adequate to meet their needs, assistance must be available for those who cannot otherwise afford the needed services. Even in the long run, of course, there will be those who must rely on the government program.

The question could be raised as to why people would establish individual accounts if the revised Medicaid program would be available to those who did not choose to set up an account. The answer is simply that people prefer to avoid having to prove their financial need to a government agency and would also want protection for the period between age 65 and 75. When the protection available through the long-term-care services proposal is added to existing cash Social Security benefits, private pensions, and Medicare, an individual will feel more self-sufficient. He can perceive his situation as one where the risk of having to depend on a means-tested public program in old age for *any* needed service will be at a minimum. Even relatively well-off aged today know that a long stay in a nursing home can soon impoverish them.

Section 3.—Because the cost of section 2 is likely to be substantial, particularly in the early years before section 1 can be fully effective, a new source of funding is proposed to meet both the federal and state share of the cost. Thus, half of the proceeds of the national lottery would be budgeted to the states to meet the costs of the new requirement, on the basis of each state's proportionate share of aged poor people. The states would receive no other federal funds for this purpose and in this sense the program would be restricted. The national lottery would be run by the federal government, contracting out functions as it found it effective to do so.

There are, of course, problems with the idea of a lottery. Public lotteries have been extensively debated in state legislatures over the last decade and only a brief statement of the major points will be made here.

Most economists agree that a public lottery is regressive since experience has shown that lower-income people tend to patronize them more than higher-income people. (George Orwell characterizes this phenomenon well in *1984*.)

Experience also suggests that income from lotteries does *not* fluctuate markedly with the business cycle and may well increase in periods of recession because more people have a reason to try to gamble their way out of a poor economic position.

The political battle around a national lottery will find two types of groups, on the negative side—organized crime and certain church groups, even though they have little else in common. Some church groups will oppose the proposal on religious and moral grounds, and organized crime because it would compete with illegal gambling. The opposition of the church groups will be open; the opposition of organized crime will not. Thus, the motives of those who argue against the proposal will be called into question.

Those states which now have lotteries may also oppose the plan, but their opposition should be muted by the fact that they would receive all the profits of the new lottery for a politically worthwhile purpose. It is possible, too, that a national lottery, earmarked for needs of the aged primarily, would be a proposal around which substantial support from the aged could be organized.

Of course, if the lottery idea is too controversial, there are other alternatives of financing which could be considered such as phasing in the new Medicaid program using present sources.

Section 4.—It is assumed that even with the individual accounts and the improved Medicaid program, it will be necessary to create resources, establish channeling agencies (community-based organizations designed to assist those in need in finding the set of services appropriate to the need), and provide services for those in need of them who are unable to pay for them and are ineligible under the Medicaid program. Thus, the proposal would budget the remaining half of the resources from the national lottery to the states on an aged-population basis to meet these more general needs.

Section 5.—This part of the overall proposal may need careful explanation, because its connection with long-term care is not so readily apparent.

The theory here is that as the aged get into their second decade, beyond age 65, they have an increasing need for a variety of supportive services, not all of which would be in the prescribed set of long-term-care benefits alluded to earlier. The increased Social Security benefits are for the purpose of making it easier for people above this age to purchase the needed services out of current income. Mechanisms for helping them find appropriate services in the community would still need to be made available.

The proposal would cost substantial amounts of money if it were to increase benefits at age 75 above the present levels and make no other changes. However, if the costs had to be kept down to gain political acceptability, benefits between ages 65 and 75 could be reduced somewhat to offset increased benefits payable at age 75. If the proposal were to have no cost, the actuaries would have to make the calculation based on life-expectancy tables. This calculation might show that a decrease of 2%–3% at age 65 could support a 5%–6% increase at age 75.

If a value-added tax is considered favorably in the future, in part as a way to adjust Social Security taxes (as discussed earlier in this paper), the cost of this proposal would be relatively modest and might be blended into the tax adjustments and other changes made at that time.

Notes

1. The theory is that a payroll tax paid by employers is inflationary because it adds directly to the cost of doing business, which most firms pass on fully (and immediately) to the consumer in increased prices for goods and services. But an increase in general revenues would be anti-inflationary because it would reduce both corporate and individual disposable income and consequently the demand for goods and services.

2. Technically, payment of the Medicare tax does not give rise to eligibility; it is working the required number of years in employment subject to the tax, whether paid or not, which gives insured status for Social Security cash benefits *and* Medicare. Yet the program is widely and correctly regarded as a system which relates contributions to eligibility.

3. Both Chairman Al Ullman (D., Ore.) of the Committee on Ways and Means of the U.S. House of Representatives and Chairman Russell Long (D., La.) of the Committee on Finance have proposed a value-added tax. Their Republican counterparts have expressed strong skepticism and opposition.

4. Part A of Medicare imposes an initial deductible on hospitalization in a set amount roughly equivalent to a day's cost of hospitalization, with a copayment (related to the deductible amount) for long hospital stays and for stays in skilled nursing facilities beyond 20 days. Part B of Medicare imposes an annual deductible amount plus a requirement that Medicare patients pay 20 percent of the amount above the deductible. In Medicaid, states are permitted to impose enrollment fees related to income for certain classes of eligibles and benefits and may impose nominal deductions, cost sharing, or similar charges for those benefits not required to be covered under the program.

5. The point is actually much more complex, of course. The definition of the units of service, and value of relationship of the listed services can greatly affect costs and patterns of utilization.

6. By capitation payment we mean simply that a set dollar payment is made to an organization, in advance, to cover the costs of providing a defined set of services over a fixed period of time to an enrolled population.

7

Cost Estimation and Long-Term-Care Policy Problems in Forecasting the Undefined

Jay Greenberg and William Pollak

Introduction
Purpose

The purpose of this paper is to derive an agenda for research in long-term care, starting from basic policy questions. Our initial intention was to write a more restricted paper, limited to identifying and describing research required to improve our capacity to forecast the cost of alternative long-term-care policies. Though narrow in scope, this focus on forecast-enabling research did not reflect narrow concerns. The most criticized aspects of this country's long-term care are its excessive reliance on institutional care and its reluctance to provide sufficient noninstitutional services. Although expanded provision of noninstitutional services is almost universally favored, it nonetheless is being effected on only a very modest scale. This slow pace is probably due to uncertainty about costs and fear that a broad noninstitutional benefit would be enormously expensive, even though advocates promise cost savings.

In this context, a paper setting forth a research plan that would dispel uncertainty about costs, though narrow, seemed important. The Congressional Budget Office, called upon to develop cost forecasts, was well aware of the need for research. They stated that "if one conclusion may be drawn" from their forecasting efforts, it was that "further research should be undertaken to assemble the data base necessary to prepare more precise estimates" (Congressional Budget Office, 1977, 2, p. 3). The CBO went on to identify several important data needs. Our intention was both to enrich the CBO's list and, more important, to go into greater detail in describing what the required research would involve; for it would have to go well beyond the collection and compilation of survey information that is suggested by the phrase "assembling the data base."

Thus our objective, initially, was an agenda that would organize research to improve our understanding of the probable cost of alternative long-term-care policies. This made the identification and categorization of policies an early priority, since the required research would depend on the types of policies that were being discussed and that had a reasonable likelihood of implementation.

However, while we were in the process of categorizing policies, issues arose that virtually compelled a broadening of focus beyond research that was directly cost related to a broader domain of research concerned with long-term care. As a result, the paper presented here is both less and more ambitious than the paper we set out to write. It is less ambitious in its effort to approximate the final product: a cookbook that would guide researchers to the data they should collect, instruments they should employ to collect them, and the particular means and models they should use in manipulating and interpreting them. It is, however, more ambitious with respect to the domain of research considered. While this broadening of scope inevitably reduces achievement relative to the issues that are raised, we hope that it produces a paper of greater value.

Approach

Long-term-care expenditures rose rapidly through the 1970s. Although estimates made in 1975 might not have accurately forecast 1980 expenditures, the forecasting task would have been manageable. Only minor long-term-care policy changes were made during the '70s, and the forecaster could have used experience and empirical relations from the early '70s as the basis for forecasts about the second half of the decade.

This procedure could not be applied to the issues addressed here. For we are concerned throughout this paper with policies that make so major a break from current practice that forecasts based on experience and relationships generated under existing programs are prohibited. Specifically, we are interested only in policies that incorporate a broadening of long-term-care benefits and that make noninstitutional services available to those who need them independent of their need for skilled care and other medical services as they are now narrowly defined.

Although many policies could do that, it is useful here to consider why such policies, which pose for some forecasters the prospect of savings, pose for others the prospect of explosive costs. The reasons are not elusive. Those who foresee reduced expenditures focus on people who were institutionalized under current policies. Since noninstitutional care for some of them would be less expensive, the provision of noninstitutional care holds out the promise of cost savings. Cost optimists tend to ignore the large number of impaired potential users of services who reside in the community and receive no care or care that is provided by a relative or friend. Cost pessimists sense that utilization of services by this latter group could conceivably impose costs that would swamp the savings produced by shifting some care from institutional to noninstitutional settings. While few are blind to the potential benefits of expanded provision of noninstitutional care, no one can accurately state what costs (positive or negative) that expansion would entail.

There obviously are two matters about which we are ignorant. One concerns the unit costs of various services, the other, utilization of those services. Although there are genuine problems in measuring and forecasting the former, they are minor relative to the problems that must be faced in forecasting the long-run growth in utilization of services that are not now provided. Forecasting the utilization of newly covered noninstitutional services is particularly treacherous because the utilization change will depend not only on a one-shot response to the price change that coverage produces but also will depend on changes that evolve slowly but significantly over time. These changes include: growing familiarity with services and service networks; declining stigma associated with using publicly financed services; altered family values and residential and helping arrangements facilitated by a noninstitutional benefit; and changes in needs for service induced by the provision of preventive services.

We are more uncertain about utilization than about unit costs. Furthermore, it is harder to gain information about utilization than about unit costs. Consequently, this paper will focus almost exclusively on utilization-related issues.

Although ignorance surrounds the cost of major changes in long-term-care policy, it is obvious that costs will depend significantly on the particulars of the policy selected. It is less obvious, but more important to our mission, to note that the information and analytic approaches required to make cost estimates also vary greatly depending on the nature of the policy. This point assumes significance when the range of long-term-care policies that are being considered is recognized. This range is apparent in articles and monographs examining policy options and/or proposing particular policies, and in memoranda within administrative agencies that lay our dimensions of long-term-care policy and complete specific policies.[1] These routinely incorporate policies as diverse as: fixed budget grants to states in place of the long-term-care elements of Medicaid; open-ended federal "insurance" approaches; shifting of all long-term-care burdens to the states in exchange for federal assumption of all Medicaid acute-care expenditures; and more modest policy shifts that would only broaden the benefit packages of the existing Medicaid and Medicare programs.

The paper is divided into three major sections. In the first section the dimensions of policy that will most likely have a major impact not only on costs but also on the nature of the cost-estimating problem are discussed. A principal theme of this paper is that the nature of a proposed policy will, to a large extent, determine the appropriate actors and activities upon which to focus cost-forecasting research. Therefore, a range of policy "caricatures" are developed. It is hoped that these caricatures will help to anchor the sometimes theoretical discussion to the realities of the decisions that we must ultimately face. The second section identifies information needs and alternative methods for obtaining information for each of the policy caricatures. The last section suggests an approach for developing a research strategy devoted to cost forecasting in long-term care.

The Policy Context of the Cost-Estimating Problem
Policy Dimensions

There are five dimensions of policy that will most likely affect the nature of the cost-estimating problem. They are as follows:

1. Nature of the prescription rules.—Under all policies, services would be prescribed and payment authorized according to some explicit or implicit rules. These rules translate the characteristics of the client (and possibly the client's family) into the particular services or resources that will be provided; with the extreme case of zero service corresponding to ineligibility. These rules, however, can vary greatly in nature. At one extreme are policies in which prescription rules or guidelines are not specified explicitly. Instead, reliance is placed on the rules implicit in professional judgment and on subjective assessments of clients' characteristics. This essentially is the procedure in our current health-care finance policies. Payment for care follows prescription decisions made by physicians on the basis of professional judgment. At the other extreme are policies in which prescription rules are specified clearly and in detail and in which the measurement of client characteristics is placed on an objective basis. These extremes are termed "flexible rule" and "rigid rule" policies, respectively. In between are policies in which guidelines are specified in order to guide and make more uniform the rules implicit in professional judgment, and policies in which rules are specified clearly but client characteristics are not objectively measured, as well as other possibilities.

Our concern here is with neither the feasibility nor the practicality of particular prescription rule options. Rather, we wish to stress that long-term-care policies similar in other respects, may differ significantly in the nature of the prescription rules that they incorporate. The choice made alone this dimension will significantly affect not only the cost of the program but also the nature of the cost-forecasting problem.

2. Nature of federal funding.—There are two basic methods of federal funding. Either a fixed budget is established at the federal level, or the federal financial commitment is open-ended. Several finance strategies would fit the former description. For example, fixed budget grants could be made to states, with each state's share determined by a formula tied to the state's characteristics. Alternatively, a fixed budget federal program might dictate a fixed amount of long-term-care capitation to be paid to providers for each person in the population over age 65.

Under any fixed budget option, other aspects of the policy are forced to accommodate to the fixed budget amount. Under open-ended funding, on the other hand, the level of expenditure accommodates to and therefore is determined by other aspects of the policy. We shall consider the role of those other aspects in shaping the estimating problem later.

3. Financial responsibility of state (and local) government.—State (and local) financial responsibility ranges from zero to 100 percent. Medicare and Medicaid both have open-ended federal funding, but they place very different financial burdens on states. Similarly, different fixed federal budget programs place different financial burdens on states. It will be argued below that not only costs but also the nature of the cost-estimating problem is very significantly affected by the amount of responsibility placed on lower levels of government.

4. Financial responsibility of clients and families.—Clients and families can be requried to pay a fraction of service costs that varies between zero and one. In actual practice, this policy dimension can become quite complex if client shares are made different for different services and for persons with different economic resources. For purposes of this discussion, it is enough to recognize that client cost shares can be set at different levels and that the level at which they are set is likely to influence utilization, private outlays, and public expenditures.

5. Organizational structure.—Many organizational matters that will influence the operation of a program will have little impact on the nature of the estimating problems that are posed. At issue here are those aspects of organization (not implicit in one of the financial dimensions above) that determine the incentives operating on the individual or unit that certifies services (or resources) for the client. Thus we are, in a sense, concerned with organizational matters that influence how well (accurately) the prescription rules will be adhered to, e.g., whether those certification decisions are made within or by entities that also produce service; whether they are made within or by entities that bear some financial burden for program services; and whether the individual or entity making certification decisions carries other responsibilities with respect to the individual.

For example, consider Medicare. Under that program physicians, who (effectively) authorize program service payments also directly produce service and additionally are case managers with respect to other services that they prescribe but do not produce. Because they function as producers and case managers, physicians may behave differently in their capacity as authorizers of third-party payments than would a service authorizer charged only with that responsibility. The producer role can give them a financial interest in their service prescriptions, while the case management role strengthens their interest in the welfare of individual clients. The organization of the Medicare program does not balance these influences with any mechanism or responsibility that would force on physicians a concern with costs. Other organizational arrangements would produce different incentives and, presumably, different prescribing behaviors.

Choices along this dimension will influence how, and how much, prescribing rules will be departed from. Because of this, policy choices along this dimension also may influence the nature of the cost-forecasting problem.

Policy "Caricatures"

The above policy dimensions are neither the only, nor, from some perspectives, the most important ones to use in defining long-term-care policy. However, they are central in shaping the cost-estimating problem and must be specified, at least implicitly, in any complete definition of long-term-care policy. Immediately below, four policy caricatures are specified in terms of choices along these dimensions. They are termed caricatures because they do not describe all aspects of a policy and because they are exceedingly spare in describing those aspects that are covered. They are presented solely as vehicles for a subsequent analysis of information needs and research directions. Policies and programs that have actually been proposed are less useful or less efficient for our purposes because they tend to incorporate irrelevant details and because incomplete specification often makes it impossible to identify the cost-estimating problems they would pose.

1. *"Rigid rules."*—Under a rigid rules policy, a specified set of prescribing rules would translate objectively measured characteristics of the individual client into the set of services (or resource amount) that would be provided. The policy presumes acceptance of some set of prescribing rules. Acceptance may reflect consensus on certain policy objectives together with technical understanding of the prescription rules required to maximize achievement of those objectives or, alternatively, may reflect consensus on prescription rules independent of technical knowledge or a consensus on objectives.

Under a policy that truly incorporates enforced rigid rules, that characteristic will dominate in determining the forecasting issues posed by the program. Choices on other policy dimensions will be dictated by the requirement that they not obstruct adherence to the rules.[2] Federal funding would have to be open-ended to ensure that all services prescribed by the rules can be funded.[3] State-local financial burdens would have to be so low that lower-level financial constraints do not limit service spending below the level determined by application of the rules. For simplicity it is assumed that the "rigid rules" policy would place no financial burdens on nonfederal levels of government. Similar reasoning applies to client cost-sharing or copayments. These are defended in health care as a means to achieve (or at least foster) allocative efficiency. They are intended to discourage consumers from using units of service whose benefits fall short of full cost by forcing users to balance perceived benefits against at least a fraction of the cost of service. However, acceptance of rigid prescription rules implies rejection of consumer assessments of service benefits. Moreover, effective implementation of rigid rules would make cost-sharing a redundant and potentially destructive constraint on use of service since it might constrain use below the level implicitly deemed optional by application of the rules.

It is assumed here that prescribing will be carried out by public entities that have no responsibilities beyond that of determining the specific services or volume of resources flowing to individual clients. The packaging and production of services are assumed to be left to other entities. The use of rigid rules and objective measures of client characteristics, however, would seem to reduce the significance of organizational structure for utilization and costs under this particular policy.

Some will regard even the idea of a "rigid rules" policy as absurd. They may view the elimination of street-level prescriber discretion as impossible and/or undesirable because of the complexity and subtlety of clients' conditions and needs for service. Therefore, it is worth noting that this hypothetical policy entered our analysis only after we noted that many expectations and assertions about long-term-care costs were based on the implicit assumption that service utilization would be determined by the application of rigid rules.

2. *Expanded and enriched Medicaid.*—Under this policy, open-ended contributions to the joint federal-state program would continue. The program would depart from present policy by mandating practices intended to broaden Medicaid coverage of noninstitutional long-term-care services. Although states can broaden coverage under existing law, few have done so. This policy would require states to: (1) cover home health, day care, respite care, homemakers, and other services normally included in the noninstitutional care package; (2) determine eligibility for these services on the basis of functional limitations independent of clients' need for skilled nursing or other medical services; (3) alter financial eligibility standards so that all persons who would be financially eligible for Medicaid nursing home care are also eligible for noninstitutional services; (4) develop a long-term-care plan incorporating designation of regional

case management organizations and the assurance of service availability in all regions; and (5) publicize the existence of the noninstitutional benefit. The policy would also incorporate an incentive for expansion of noninstitutional care by raising the federal share on such services to a level significantly higher than the normal federal Medicaid share to the state.

Because this policy is specified as a modification of Medicaid, the implicit client "cost-sharing" terms under Medicaid would be continued, except for modifications required to make them consistent with the modified financial eligibility standards. Although payment for services now is generally certified by independent physicians using professional standards, states would be free to adopt more rigid standards and to implement them through certifications carried out within the state Medicaid program.

3. *Fixed budget/state grants.*—Under this policy, a fixed federal budget would be established legislatively and each state would be allocated a share of the total determined by formula. The grant would replace all federal Medicaid payments for long-term care, and states would be required to match the federal grant with an amount at least equal to their former expenditures for long-term care under Medicaid. This policy substitutes for the rigidity of fixed prescription rules a rigidity of expenditure amounts. Under rigid rules, expenditures must be open-ended so that funding can conform to the service implications of the rules. Correspondingly, if federal allocations are fixed, states must be given considerable autonomy so that their policies (prescribing behavior, state contributions in excess of any required state match, and so forth) will yield an excess of expenditures over state contributions that conforms to their fixed federal allocation. Beyond its minimal required contribution, each state must have freedom to establish the prescription rules, cost-sharing arrangement, and organizational structure that are most appropriate to its unique needs.

4. *A new Medicare benefit: "Medicare Part C."*—This policy benefit would supplement most benefits of Medicare parts A and B and would replace the home health benefits of those parts. It would cover the standard package of noninstitutional services: home health, homemaker, personal care, social and nutrition services, and day and respite care. It would, however, not only extend the benefit to some services not covered in parts A and B, but also would extend eligibility to those whose need is unrelated to an acute illness or injury and to those without a need for skilled care.

Other dimensions of the program would parallel existing Medicare practice. The program would be funded entirely out of federal funds and would incorporate the current cost-sharing terms of Medicare. Certification might be by independent physicians, or PSRO and other current forms of utilization review might perform internal certification by the application of rigid rules.

Information Needs and Alternative Methods for Obtaining Information

In this section, the different information needs associated with each of the policy caricatures are discussed, and alternative methods of obtaining the information are considered. Underlying policy objectives will emerge as key factors in defining the specifics of each policy and hence in defining the nature of its cost-estimating problem. The relative length of the various subsections varies substantially. This variation is more a reflection of the state of our knowledge, than it is of the importance of the item.

Rigid Rules

Even if it were unattainable in practice, a policy incorporating adherence to rigid rules would have heuristic value. A rigid rules policy fosters recognition of those estimating problems that survive even when there is a high level of control over utilization. Additionally, centrally imposed rigidity focuses attention on information about treatment effects, broadly viewed. Such information would seem essential in legitimating the imposition of rigid rules. This information also is important under more flexible, centrally directed policies.

Utilization of various long-term-care services can be seen as determined in two stages: the stage which gets the client into the program and the stage incorporating all those decisions that determine utilization once the client is engaged in the program. A rigid rules policy would sharply differentiate the mechanisms operating in those two stages. Consequently, the approach appropriate to estimating utilization determination in the first stage is largely inappropriate to estimating utilization determination in the second stage.

Seeking Service.—As was discussed above, to estimate the cost of a policy based upon rigid rules, it is important to recognize that the ultimate quantities of services consumed are determined not only by the set of established prescribing rules, but also by how many people seek care. That is, the nature of the rigid rules determines the quantities of service and hence the cost of caring for a particular "type" of long-term-care recipient. However, in order to estimate the cost of the program, it is necessary also to determine how many of each "type" of potential recipient will seek care. Thus, one of the tasks in estimating the cost of the program is the estimation of the number and "types" of potential recipients who will seek care under the new program.

A useful way to approach this problem is to ask, "what is the probability that certain 'types' of people will seek care?"—where "type" is defined in terms of those variables that will ultimately be used to determine service quantities (i.e., the variables that constitute the prescribing rules). If the probabilities of particular "types" of persons seeking care are estimated, then the expected numbers of each type of client can be established. This information, coupled with the prescribing formula, can be used to estimate the total quantities of service that can be expected to be required in a particular period of time for a particular catchment area.

The question then is what kind of procedure for generating and analyzing information will provide reliable and valid estimates of these probabilities and resulting expected numbers of program applicants? We initially identified three methods for obtaining these data:

1. A social-epidemiological survey coupled with preference survey.
2. The use of past or ongoing long-term-care demonstration projects in conjunction with a social-epidemiological survey of the catchment area.
3. New demand experiments in conjunction with a social-epidemiological survey of the catchment area.

In order to evaluate the potential of each method, we also list seven elements that will affect the reliability and validity of these estimates.

1. *Prescribing rules must be established.*—There are two reasons why the prescribing rules should be established prior to the beginning of the study. First, the prescribing rules themselves are, to a large extent, the intervention. If we are to understand the results of the experiment or program, we must know what the program was. Second, the nature of the prescribing rules might influence care-seeking behavior.

2. *Definition of the catchment area.*—In order to establish rates of utilization, it is necessary first to establish the exact geographic boundaries of the catchment area(s).

3. *Estimation of the total number of potential recipients living in the catchment area.*—Ultimately we are interested in estimating the probability of each "type" of recipient's seeking care. Therefore, it is essential that estimates of the total number of each "type" of potential recipient be generated. Since "type" refers to the variables used in the prescribing formula, the nature of the needed denominator data will be determined by the variables in that formula. However, regardless of which prescribing rule is followed, it seems apparent that these types of data will not be available from existing secondary sources.[4] Therefore, some form of social-epidemiological survey of the catchment area will be required.

4. *Perceptions about the demonstration projects benefit package must be similar to those about the new policy if it were implemented.*—In general this implies that if the experiences that generate the data are to have external validity, then perceptions about the benefits of the demonstration project must be similar to the perceptions of the benefit package of the new policy. It is important to note that it is the *perception* of benefits that is important and not the actual benefits. Below, we will discuss the important role that time will play in shaping people's perceptions as to the legitimacy of the program.

5. *Referral networks and the types of people referred must be similar to those that will emerge as a result of the enactment of the new policy.*— Most people do not self-refer to long-term-care demonstration projects or ongoing long-term-care programs. They are usually referred to the program by information and referral services, providers, or family and friends. It therefore is essential that the referral pattern used to channel people into the demonstration project be similar to the pattern that will develop upon the maturity of the new policy. Aside from the legitimating role that time plays, the nature and type of promotion must also be similar.

6. *Availability of, and eligibility for, alternative programs must be similar to those that will be available at the time the new policy is established.*—The number and types of people seeking the benefits of a particular program will be partially determined by the availability of alternative programs that they perceive to be close substitutes for that program. Therefore, either it is necessary to maintain a similar mix of alternatives under both the demonstration program and the ongoing policy, or the analyst must be able to estimate the degree of substitutions that can be expected. For example, if under a demonstration project a potential client can receive personal care or chore services through a different public or voluntary program, then he will have a lower probability of seeking these benefits under the demonstration program. Now suppose that part of the new policy is to do away with or modify eligibility for these other programs. One could reasonably hypothesize that the demand for the services under the new policy would be substantially greater than the demand for the same set of services under the demonstration program.

7. *Supply must not be a binding constraint.*—When services are bought and sold in markets, the single market price and utilization are jointly determined; demand (the quantity clients want to use) is equal to supply, and people are able to use all that they want to at the market price. However, subsidization of service use is at the core of long-term-care policy. The price paid by clients is lower than the price paid to providers. Price becomes an instrument of policy rather than the product of market forces, so that an equilibrium where supply and demand are unequal is possible. What supply will actually be, and what relation it will bear to

demand, will be largely determined by underlying cost conditions interacting with the price that is determined by reimbursement policy.

This policy can be managed in several ways. For example, reimbursement policy can be managed so that providers are induced to supply quantities that approximate the quantities clients demand (want) at the subsidy price. Utilization then will be equal to and determined by demand. Reimbursement policies that cause supply to accommodate to subsidized demand and that enable utilization to equal demand will be referred to as "accommodative" reimbursement policies.

Alternatively, in pursuit of cost control or other objectives, reimbursement (and other, possibly direct-control, policies) may be managed in a way that causes providers to supply a substantially smaller quantity than clients want at the subsidy price. Since clients can use only services that are supplied, utilization in this instance would be less than demand—indeed would be independent of demand forces—and would be determined by supply. Reimbursement (or some other policy) that produces excess demands will be termed "restrictive."

Estimates of demand can be based only on experience generated under "accommodative" policies; that is, only under policies that remove supply as a constraint on utilization. This has implications for forecast-enabling research regardless of approach.[5]

With these seven necessary conditions in mind, we shall briefly examine the likely usefulness of each of the three methods of obtaining data on seeking behavior.

Social—epidemiological survey coupled with a preference survey.—One method of obtaining the needed estimate of service-seeking behavior would be to develop a social-epidemiological survey and couple it with a preference survey. As discussed above, to be useful, the data items collected through the epidemiological survey should be the same as those items that make up the prescribing formula. In turn, the items or variables that constitute the prescribing formula should be based upon the underlying policy objectives. If properly designed and carried out, the social-epidemiological survey can provide the needed denominator data for predefined catchment areas. Issues here would have to do with developing an appropriate sampling methodology, drawing an adequate sample size, and the use or development of a reliable and valid survey instrument.

In contrast, the design and implementation of the preference survey present formidable obstacles. First, it is not even clear who should be sampled. Should potential recipients be sampled, families of potential recipients, doctors, discharge planners, or personnel at information and referral services? That is, since there is little information available about who the decision makers really are, it becomes difficult to develop a meaningful sampling frame.

Second, there is little evidence to suggest that answers to questions such as "What would you do if...?" have much predictive validity with regard to how the person will actually behave if actually confronted with that situation. Furthermore, even if statements of preferences were predictive of behavior, it could be only in the very short run. Therefore, these estimates could not be relied upon for long-run or equilibrium demand projections.

Finally, this approach cannot possibly deal adequately with the issues of changing availability of alternative programs or the effects of relaxed supply constraints.

The use of past or ongoing long-term-care demonstration projects in conjunction with a social-epidemiological survey of the catchment area.—Given the inherent problems of preference or opinion surveys, an alternative might be to use data from past or ongoing long-term-care demonstration projects. Once again, these data would be used in conjunction with a social-epidemiological survey of the catchment area. This approach has the advantage of using actual rather than proposed behavior, and the incremental costs of this approach to estimation would be relatively small. Furthermore, the lead time between inception and results would be considerably shorter than a new demand experiment (discussion below). However, there are several fundamental problems with past and current long-term-care demonstration projects that do not augur well for their use in making demand projections.

First, most past and current long-term-care demonstration projects do not present well-established prescribing rules. For the most part these projects use "clinical judgments" as a mechanism for prescribing services to participants.[6] Related to this is the fact that the target population and the actual population served by these projects differed across projects and may not conform to the desired target population that would be specified by the prescribing rules.

Because of long start-up delays and implementation difficulties, many of these projects provided services for only a relatively short period of time (usually less than 36 months). Therefore, this experience cannot be used to examine long-run demand or supply adjustment behaviors.

Finally, and most important of all, these projects were not designed to be demand studies. Consequently, target case loads were established. If and when these quotas were filled, no new clients were permitted (unless the case load dropped below the quota). Waiting lists from those projects that met their care quotas will not be very useful in estimating potential demand, because assessment data were often not obtained until the potential client was off the unit list and became an actual client, and because there is no way to estimate how many potential clients were not referred to the project as a result of a long waiting list. It, therefore, seems doubtful that past or current demonstration projects can shed much light on the issue of potential demand.

This would suggest the need to consider the development of a new set of demonstration projects—projects designed specifically to estimate demand or expected utilization rates.

New demand experiments in conjunction with a social-epidemiological survey of the catchment area.—At the risk of greatly oversimplifying a very complex process, a demand experiment would need to go through the following broadly defined tasks or steps:

1. Through research or other means, develop prescription rules.
2. Develop research design and instrumentation.
3. Design and carry out a social-epidemiological survey to estimate the number of potential clients.
4. Develop an organizational structure and choose the site of the lead agency or organization.
5. Establish reimbursement mechanisms.
6. Establish a referral network.
7. Establish a relationship with providers.
8. Take in, assess, and service clients.
9. Analyze.
10. Phase out or adopt the policy.

If properly designed, implemented, and analyzed, a demand experiment, as outlined above, would have a good chance of establishing meaningful estimates of demand. However, to be done correctly it would have to be quite large and of long duration. As a result it would be very expensive.

The nature of the inquiry is such that within a specified catchment area the sampling of potential clients would not be feasible. Recall that the basic objective of the experiment is to estimate what proportion of the eligible population in a given area will either self-refer or be referred to the program. Therefore, the way the natural referral network works will be a key determining factor of demand. If referral sources are asked to refer only a certain percentage of their clients or if only a certain percentage of the eligible self-referrals are accepted into the program, this will clearly have an impact on their behavior, thus biasing the estimate of demand.

This need for a "saturation" experiment is in sharp contrast to the requirements of other social experiments such as the negative income tax experiments, the National Health Insurance experiments, and the demand elements of the housing allowance experiments. In these three cases, the object of the inquiry was to examine the behavior of participants *after* they had entered the program. Their postadmission behavior was then compared with that of groups of individuals who did not receive program benefits. In these cases randomized samplings made sense. However, the nature of the long-term-care demand experiment under rigid rules is not to investigate client behavior *after* entrance into the program, but rather to estimate how many of them will enter the program.

Therefore, within a given catchment area, the number of recipients is likely to be large. Furthermore, the nature of the local delivery system, attitudes of local providers, and social, economic, and ethnic makeup of the residents of a catchment area will probably affect demand; we can expect large variations in demand *across* catchment areas. This being the case, a sizable number of sites would be required to make accurate national projections.

Not only would the experiment need to be large, but it would also need to be of rather long duration. First, the initial set of prescribing rules must be developed. Second, due to the complex nature of the system level of intervention, the period of time devoted to developing, planning, and implementing the intervention will need to be rather lengthy. Finally, and most important, since what we are seeking are long-run or equilibrium demand projections, the intervention itself must operate over an extended period of time. It must operate long enough for information to be disseminated, referral networks developed or adjusted, and attitudes and beliefs altered. That is, the program must gain legitimacy among planners, providers, professionals, and potential recipients and their families. Once legitimacy is established, the various actors must be given enough time to adjust their behavior. It is the measurement of behavior, after this adjustment process, that is desired. How long will all of this take? Obviously, nobody knows. Nevertheless, it would seem unreasonable to assume that the entire process, from design to data analysis, could be accomplished in less than ten years (and probably closer to fifteen years).

Thus far in this section, we have explored three alternative ways of estimating the potential demand for services under a rigid-rules long-term-care policy. Two of the three (preference surveys and the use of data from past studies) have been rejected because they are not likely to provide useful results. The third alternative, a demand experiment, while promising in its ability to generate the needed data, will require a huge amount of resources and will probably require at least a decade. Are there any other methods of obtaining the needed information?

As will be discussed in the concluding section of this paper, an alternative to a formal demonstration strategy would be the incremental implementation of rigid rules policy. The phased implementation of the policy could be used to generate demand data, and these data could then be used to make mid-course corrections.

Utilization by those who enter the system.—Estimating services' utilization for those who enter the system raises issues that depend to a large degree on the nature of the prescription rules. Here it is assumed that the rules translate client characteristics into a specific service package and that clients will accept the full prescribed package. Other types of prescription rules and behaviors are possible, but these are particularly useful in identifying estimating problems.

Given the mix of people estimated to enter the program the existence of rigid rules greatly simplifies the second stage of estimating utilization. For, applying the rigid rules to the estimated mix of clients mechanically yields estimates of the services that will initially be prescribed and used. The problem assumes more than mechanical complexity only because of the need to estimate the changes over time in client characteristics that will call forth changing service prescriptions. Implicit in appeals for expanded preventive care is the notion that services provided now, through effects on clients and informal caretakers, will reduce the future need for formal care. If this notion is correct, estimates of utilization over time, even under a regime of rigid rules, will require information not only on the mix of people entering the care system, but also on the effects of services on the needs of clients and their informal supports.

Rationalizing prescription rules: information needs.—Mention of the needs trajectories of clients and families suggests a different range of issues that merit separate attention. The universal imposition of uniform prescribing rules can be defended as fostering horizontal equity, cost control, and other possible objectives. However, the practice would gain in legitimacy if the particular rules had some rationale.

One rationale would exist if the needs associated with various conditions were so apparent that virtually all observers would agree on the service mixes appropriate to particular conditions. Kutza (chap. 4, p. 126, above) notes the error in this expectation. "Identification of a functional limitation does not directly translate into a service need. For example, a person may have difficulty walking around. A response to that problem can take various forms—a wheelchair, a walker, a cane, better shoes, podiatry services." A number of studies empirically document the wide variance in services that different professionals will prescribe for the same individual when free to use their own professional judgment.[7]

In the absence of ad hoc consensus on the services appropriate to a particular condition, the imposition of rigid rules would seem defensible only if particular rules could somehow be shown to be "best." It is critical here to note that any approach to the identification of "best" prescription rules would require (1) a specification of the objectives of policy and (2) identification of the technical relation between services provided and the client (and family) outcomes that are the objectives of policy. These matters have been raised in the context of policies that incorporate rigid rules. However, if rigid rules are for any reason unattainable or undesirable in practice, then thought and information on objectives and service-outcome relations are needed to guide and rationalize the prescription of services under flexible rules policies that permit the exercise of professional judgment. The discussion that follows thus has relevance beyond the rigid rules context in which it arises.[28]

Objectives.—Our intent in this section is to present a short list of objectives that will capture more people's concerns when advocating public support for long-term care and when deliberating over the particulars of long-term-care policy. The following three objectives are inclusive but not exhaustive. Although different words are usually used, most objectives in the standard litany either approximate objectives listed here or represent an objective that is instrumental in achieving one of them.

1. *Compensate for "tough breaks":* Long-term-care policy exists primarily to compensate people who suffer chronic impairments for the personal and financial costs of their condition. To the question, why should the public sector shoulder responsibility for long-term care, one response is: because society has an obligation to compensate those who by chance are the unfortunate sufferers of chronic impairments. If set within a social insurance context, pursuit of the compensation objective would imply equal (gross and) net (of coinsurance) benefits for people in different economic situations.[9]

If the objective of policy is simply to compensate people, benefits in the form of financial grants are suggested. Beneficiaries should be free to use their benefit to purchase institutional or noninstitutional services of their own choosing—except in instances where the beneficiary is demonstrably incompetent as a consumer and has no informed responsible helper to assist.

2. *Maintenance of minimum standard of living:* Society today assures virtually all its members a standard of living above some socially defined minimum. Long-term-care policy exists to make possible the maintenance of that minimum standard for persons whose impairments increase its cost and complexity. Long-term-care policy in this view is an extension of income maintenance policy. Benefits should flow only to those with inadequate resources and only in the amount required to supplement individuals' resources to a level that meets the (minimum) cost of living associated with their impairments.

Two views may be adopted with respect to the prescription rules implied by this objective. In one view, society should seek only to assure that all have sufficient resources to meet the cost of the minimum standard. In that view, the prescription rules need specify only the resource amounts appropriate to each level of impairment. In a second view, society has in mind specific living standard elements and seeks to assure, particularly with respect to impairment-related needs, that those living standard minima are maintained; adequate nutrition, housing, personal and environmental hygiene, and so forth. In this view prescription rules would have to specify not only resource amounts, but also the specific services whose provision will ensure maintenance of the standard of living defined in detail.

3. *Minimization of decline:* the objective of long-term-care policy is to minimize decline and to foster improvement or rehabilitation where that is possible. This objective can relate to one dimension of client condition or to some mix of several dimensions. Thus the characteristic of concern might be physical functioning, instrumental functioning, or functioning in social roles. But, however viewed, the objective of policy would be to keep the impaired from becoming more impaired and to reduce impairments when possible.

Thus, in this view, the dictates of another objective determine the distribution of benefits among persons, but minimization of decline is the objective that determines the particular services provided to each individual. For example, compensation requirements could determine the volume of resources allocated to an individual; but in order to minimize decline these resources would be used to provide the package of services that best preserves the client's social, physical, and/or mental functioning. This blending of the compensation and decline-minimization objectives would require sacrificing the freedom-of-choice aspect associated above with the compensation objective.

In the second light, minimization of decline can be viewed as a global objective that should govern the disposition of resources among individuals as well as the use of resource amounts assigned to particular individuals. In this view, limited long-term-care resources should flow most to persons on whom they will have the greatest impact. If resources will have little effect on an individual's condition over time, then they should flow to another person who will be more affected by them.

Global application of this objective might not be as heartless or harmful as this presentation suggests. Some minimum living standard is required for all people if lack of nutrition, heat, hygiene, medical care, and social contact is not to induce decline. The objective of minimizing decline, therefore, would assure all persons some minimum standard of living. However, in allocating services above that minimum, global application of this objective would target services on those who can be most affected by them.

The reader may think that the differences between these objectives are subtle and that one can easily settle for comfortable simultaneous pursuit of two or three. The fallacy of that notion is apparent if the allocation implications of the minimization-of-decline and compensation objectives are contrasted. Many persons whose impairments merit "compensation" would be denied service if minimization-of-decline were the objective because their decline is unresponsive to service.

Our concern here, however, is not with the very real policy implications of objectives. Rather we wish to identify the information that is needed in prescribing for different objectives and to examine various mechanisms for obtaining that information.

Information needs and methods for obtaining information for rational prescribing under specified objectives.—Prescribing rules can be considered rational only in the context of some objective(s). For this reason three plausible objectives for long-term-care policy were presented. However, even in the context of a particular objective, prescribing rules are rational only if they represent the set of rules that maximize achievement of the objective. Consequently, identification of prescribing rules also requires technical information about how various services affect the achievement of objectives for clients with various characteristics—that is, technical information on the service-outcome relationship.

This makes it evident that the technical information required to inform the prescribing decision also depends on the objective(s) selected. Thus, a different kind of information about the impact of service is required if the objective of service is the minimization of decline rather than simple compensation for the misfortune of impairments. This in turn implies that methods for obtaining information will differ among the various objectives. Information needs related to the service-outcome relation, therefore, are considered within the context of the three objectives distinguished above.

Minimization of decline.—Certain services provided to certain clients and their family units retard the decline (and possibly foster the improvement) of the client's condition. Other services may not have that effect. Rules (rigid or flexible) that allocate service so as to minimize decline of the chronically ill require for their identification information on the impact of various services on the decline of individuals with various functional and medical characteristics.

These are two interrelated tasks with regard to research on the effects of long-term-care services on decline trajectories. The first is to estimate the impact various sets of services have on client decline for each "type" of client. The second is to estimate which "types" of client benefit most from services—where, again, benefits are measured in terms of maximizing improvements or minimizing decline. Coupled with cost data, these results would lead to the identification of cost-effective treatment modalities as well as the groups of clients for whom these services are most cost effective.

In designing a research project to address the above question, particular attention must be paid to the following issues:

1. *Domain of concern:* The starting point for this study should be a clear articulation of what dimensions of health and functioning are to be considered.

2. *Selection or development of measurement instruments:* It is essential that reliable and valid client assessment instruments be selected or developed. Futhermore, it is important that these instruments be sensitive to change.

3. *Development of meaningful client grouping:* A methodology must be adopted or developed that allows for the initial grouping of clients. These groups should be predictive of overall resource consumption and should have meaning to clinician and care managers. Furthermore, to keep the size of the experiment reasonable, there should be a manageable number of groupings. The development of meaningful groupings will not be an easy task, but it is an essential element of the research.

4. *Substantial within-group service variation:* If meaningful differences in outcomes (rates of decline) are hoped for, then the experiment must provide for substantial variation in types and quantities of services within each client group. In developing these service packages, it will probably be useful to use both a panel of experts and any relevant data from past long-term-care demonstration projects that might be obtained. Not only should the types and quantities of the services be varied, but the target of the intervention should also be varied. In particular, the amounts and kinds of support provided to family and friends should also be varied.

5. *Duration:* Care must be given to ensure that the period of the intervention is sufficiently long so that the impacts of the interventions can be felt.

6. *Phasing:* The above-mentioned tasks are by no means trivial. Proper instrumentation, client grouping, and service variation will require careful study. It is quite possible that no adequate methodologies will emerge. It would, therefore, be wise to separate the project into two phases—a feasibility/development phase and an experimental phase. Only after the initial design has been carefully scrutinized by long-term-care research experts, should the experimental phase be initiated.

It is important to emphasize that this type of study is very similar to a medical-clinical trial and is not a provider or organizational demonstration project. That is, the purpose of the experiment is to test technological relationships and not organizational or political issues. Therefore, these studies should be conducted in and by well-established long-term-care research organizations. Furthermore, it would be unwise to conduct this research as part of a demonstration project that was testing system-level interventions, such as new organizational or financial arrangements.

Minimum standard of living.—As discussed above, a second possible objective stems from the notion that society may wish to ensure people an acceptable standard of living. When impairments occur, the cost of maintaining that standard is increased; at least by the cost of services that substitute for functions formerly carried out by the individual. Compensation in this view would consist of offsetting the increment to living costs associated with various impairments. Identification of those costs involves a strong subjective element that is best acknowledged in specifying information needs. Information required to effect "compensation of living costs" is a set of informed social judgments about the levels of cost increments associated with various impairments.

Two plausible approaches for obtaining this information are suggested here. Under one, a group would be convened for the purpose of developing informed judgments. Several techniques can be used to foster the evolution of consensus, but two types of information would be given to the group to increase the validity of outcomes. First, the group would be familiarized with the standard of living provided to the unimpaired by income maintenance programs. This would include information on the dollar benefits of those programs and the physical and social conditions attainable with those benefits. Second, experts could provide information on specific impairments, the needs they create and the services that can address those needs. With this as input, possibly supplemented by information on complimentary minimum standards of nutrition, personal hygiene, clean environment, socialization, and related matters, the group could seek consensus on the services that would be required to maintain a minimum living standard.

A second, rather different procedure might make less abstract the derivation of standards-maintaining service packages appropriate to various impairments. Under this approach a demonstration service program would be established with the primary objective of establishing a relationship between impairment level and service package. Case managers would be told that their objective in assigning services was to maintain their clients at a minimum living standard defined in terms suggested above: eating properly, living in a clean place, seeing enough other people, and so forth. Case managers would have open-ended funding with which to purchase appropriate services, be encouraged to maintain good information on their clients' situation, and have small case loads that are consistent with the project's objective. A major feature of the project would be continuous review of the service assignments of different case managers, the comparison of service assignments of different case managers, and the feedback of information to case managers to foster convergence of assignments toward consensus. Standards-maintaining service packages would be those toward which practice converged in this context.

Compensation for tough breaks.—It is important to note that the minimum standard of living criterion was established external to the individual. That is, it was a social judgment that placed the minimum standard at SSI (or whatever). In the case of compensation for tough breaks, it is individuals' subjective evaluation of the "psychic" cost to them of their impairments that is to be measured. This approach assumes that, in concept, people can place a dollar cost on the amount of suffering their impairments have caused.

One method that could be used to estimate what the levels of compensation would have to be is to ask groups of unimpaired persons how much they would be willing to pay to prevent the onset of a particular impairment or set of impairments. This approach would be identical to that used by Acton and others in evaluating the subjective value of lifesaving programs.

While the willingness to pay concept is interesting and may even be conceptually correct, numerous practical and measurement problems may prevent its application. Indeed, according to Acton:

> The principal practical problems with the willingness to pay procedure for benefit estimation is that developing accurate assessments of individuals' willingness to pay is difficult and expensive and the validity of published attempts to apply various estimations-techniques is questionable. Furthermore, the extent to which estimates of a particular population group's willingness to pay for a particular safety enhancing project can be applied to other groups and other types of projects is unknown.[10]

Expanded and Enriched Medicaid

In estimating the cost of an expanded and enriched Medicaid policy, it is useful to focus on the matter of state control. Even if a broader service package, outreach, and other matters are federally mandated, states will retain substantial control over the level of long-term-care expenditures. There is some evidence that wide variations among states in rates of nursing home utilization reflect variations in bed availability that are, in turn, determined by state reimbursement practices. Reimbursement policy, thus, is one means through which states can exercise control over current and future outlays under the Medicaid program. But there are other ways for states to control the net impact of the policy on their Medicaid expenditures, if the policy tends significantly to increase long-term-care expenditures. For example, compensating reductions may be made in other areas. Those who think that mandated benefits and open-ended federal funding remove Medicaid expenditure levels from state control should ponder cross-state variations in per capita and per recipient Medicaid expenditure. These variations suggest that in the long run, if not in the short run, states do somehow exert considerable influence on Medicaid expenditures.

If the object is to estimate federal expenditures under this policy, an extreme view would argue, in light of state control, that the problem has relatively little to do with the specifics of client characteristics and client and professional behavior in the area of long-term care. Rather the issue is one of forecasting state behavior when the federal government will share open-endedly in financing a new range of services for a specified population. Even in the less extreme view that we would favor, a federal effort to estimate the federal budgetary impact of this policy should focus substantially on state behaviors, recognizing that those may be somewhat affected by the specific demand pressures generated by the policy.

This is not a trivial shift in perspective. It implies that information needed to estimate the federal cost of this policy is information about state behaviors under other state/federal policies with similar financial structures rather than information about demands, needs, or other matters specific to long-term care.

In order to predict state behavior it is important first to examine "state preferences." The examination of preferences reveals two very different processes that states go through. Both of these will have an important impact on the federal cost of an expanded Medicaid program. First, as has been well documented elsewhere, states will most likely attempt to maximize the amount of net federal revenues that they can receive.[11] That is, if given the option, states would prefer to spend federal dollars rather than state dollars. Second, through the legislative process, states make resource allocation decisions to various programs and activities. The result of the "pulling and hauling" process is a set of decisions that determine the level of state spending and the distribution of state spending among various programs. Therefore, any attempt to estimate the federal cost of an expanded Medicaid program should begin by first examining the implications of these two phenomena.

As indicated above, part of the cost to the federal government of an expanded Medicaid program will be nothing more than a redistribution of the cost of current programs from state and local governments to the federal government. The magnitude of this shift will be a function of the types of services that are added to the Medicaid program and current state

spending on these services for the Medicaid eligible population. Therefore, what is needed is first an articulation of what new services will be
added or what old restrictions will be removed. Second, state and local
health and social service cost reporting should be examined so that an
estimate of current state and local spending on these services, for this
population, can be estimated. Unfortunately, given the status of state and
local social service cost-reporting systems, accurate estimates will be
difficult and for some states impossible to obtain. Nevertheless, rough
estimates are possible. For example, in Minnesota, if a new expanded
long-term care Medicaid component included chore services, adult day
care, home-delivered meals, congregate dining, homemaking service, and
transportation services, and if current Medicaid eligibility was maintained, then the state would be in a position to shift the cost of approximately 4.5 million dollars of services to the federal government (assuming
no change in state matching rates). This estimate is based upon data from
the states' Comprehensive Annual Service Plan, the Social Service Reporting System, and interviews with Minnesota Department of Public
Welfare personnel.[12]

In addition to estimating the potential redistributive effects of the new
policy, we must also try and estimate how much states will be willing to
allocate to this expanded program. Possible methods to be explored
would include examining and modeling past budgetary decisions and
trends, and identifying and interviewing key local political actors. The
methods used by Richard Nathan and associates to evaluate the fiscal
impacts of the Community Development Block Grant Program may be a
useful starting point.[13] Since the state is clearly a prime decision maker
with regard to expenditures under the Medicaid program, if adequate
models for predicting state expenditure behavior cannot be developed,
accuracy in forecasting the cost of an expanded Medicaid program cannot
be expected.

To the degree that there is interest in a policy of this type, the research
directions implied above are appropriate for federal cost-estimating
needs. However, it may be argued that the line of reasoning again is
excessively parochial in its single-minded concern with the *federal* cost-
estimating problem. Even though states may be able to control expenditures, they presumably would like to be able to estimate the costs they
would encounter were they to use their newly available long-term-care
funds in different ways. This view is reasonable. However, the policies
that states would be choosing among would be policies that are, in their
essentials, close to one or another of the options considered. As a conse-
quence, the information they would need for estimating their costs is
information that is considered in one of the other sections.

Fixed Federal Budget/State Grants

Given our preoccupation with the problems of estimating costs, it is worth noting and even emphasizing the most obvious of points: from a federal perspective a fixed budget program could eliminate uncertainty about federal outlays and eliminate the need to forecast federal long-term-care expenditures. This, of course, is a patently parochial federal view since states might not regard their outlays as fixed and certainly would retain interest in the cost implications of establishing their (autonomous) programs in various ways. However, it can be noted again that state problems in estimating their costs would correspond, at least conceptually, to the cost-estimating problems faced by the federal government under one of the other policies considered above and below. For this reason they are not separately examined here.

Although fixed budget state grants would eliminate problems of forecasting federal outlays, they would not eliminate a federal interest in costs or in forecasting other aspects of the program. It is worth briefly considering the nature of those interests and the information needs they create. The discussion focuses separately on information needs related to the establishment of state grants and information needs related to broader aspects of state grant programs operation.

Establishment of state grants.—If state shares of a budget are to be determined by formula, the formula should be as reasonable as possible. Two approaches are distinguished, a purist approach and an ad hoc approach. Under a purist approach, the federal government would have in mind prescribing rules consistent with some objective(s) such as those discussed above. State shares would then be based on the application of the prescribing rules to the state's population as it appears in survey data describing it, as much as possible in terms of the characteristics used in prescribing rules. Information needs implied by this purist approach are apparent. First, in its most rarified form the prescribing rules would be rationalized—implying information needs already discussed. Even if prescribing rules were arbitrarily established, information needs remain. Ideally, survey data would be obtained describing the population in terms of the variables employed in the prescribing rules. Failing that, it would be useful to obtain empirical estimation of the relation between easily measured population characteristics on which data are regularly available (age, sex, family status, rural vs. urban residence, occupation, and so forth), and the occurrence of the various impairments and medical conditions that dictate service provision under the selected prescription rules. These would permit state allocations more consistent with prescribing intentions than direct use of data on such variables as age, sex, and family status.

It is difficult to anticipate the directions a more ad hoc approach to a state grant formula might take but less difficult to specify information that could improve the quality of the effort. First, survey information on the incidence of impairments would, once again, be of use—as would studies on the relation between easily measured characteristics and the incidence of long-term-care need. Long-term-care utilization and expenditures vary greatly across states. Improved information on the determinants of these variations under the existing open-ended federal-state Medicaid program would seem important, if a fixed budget program is equitably to be put in its place. Upper midwest states tend to make unusually great use of nursing home care—a pattern that might be attributed to climate (harsh winters), low population density, and high out-migration of younger generations; or alternatively the pattern might be due to more liberal funding of nursing home care. It should be apparent that better understanding of how these forces operate in determining current state expenditures would be helpful in deciding the degree to which current federal assistance (through Medicaid) should be replicated or overruled under a formula approach.

State grant program: Other (major) issues.—A state grant approach has obvious attractions. It would permit a possible broadening of the boundaries of long-term care while maintaining fiscal control, at least at the federal level. The establishment of a reasonable grant formula is one concern posed by such a program—but it is less vexing than the question of what policies states might follow were the policy put in place. This is hardly a trivial issue or one that can be addressed with great confidence before the fact. Nonetheless, if a state grant program for long-term care is an option up for serious consideration, these questions deserve more attention. Cost estimation becomes a minor or trivial concern at the federal level under state block grants and should be replaced by very serious efforts to forecast the policies that states might implement were the policy world to shift so significantly. These efforts would be concerned both with the impact of grants on state spending on long-term-care services (as opposed to other services toward which grant funds might flow) and with their impact on the form that long-term-care programs might take. In a recent paper, Hudson enumerates several issues that must be carefully examined in the context of the development of a long-term-care block grant program. Among those issues he identifies are the need to develop means for ensuring that:
1. Persons currently being served cannot be dropped from the system.
2. Current service options cannot be pressured out of existence because they belong to programs being folded into the block grant system.

3. Mechanisms are in place which assure acceptable quality of care.
4. The federal government has some meaningful way of enforcing the legislative and regulatory provisions contained in federal legislation.

Whether these issues become problems under a block grant approach is, of course, a function of how the states behave in the face of the program. Thus, once again, research should be focused on likely state behavior in implementing the program. Short of suggesting, as we did in the section on Medicaid, that past state behavior be examined, the authors are not in a position to recommend a specific research strategy to help address these questions.

Medicare Part C

Medicare part C would make a broadened home care package available to a population much larger than the population now eligible for home health benefits under Medicare parts A and B. Services would be prescribed and provided under financial and organizational arrangements similar to those used for acute medical services. However, the change in benefits and eligibility would be sufficiently great to make inappropriate any forecasting of costs based on relationships observed under the current Medicare program. It is assumed here that reimbursement policy will be accommodative so that utilization will, in the long run, be determined by user demand decisions filtered through the prescribing and certifying behaviors of physicians, rather than by a supply constraint.

This is potentially the most expensive of the options considered here; expensive in its benefit package, in the open-endedness of its funding, and in its reliance on independent practitioners for certification decisions based on professional judgment. Of course, it is possible that the program would evolve toward more standardization of prescribing rules and greater control over prescribing behavior; for example, through preadmission screening, prior authorization, or other measures. If standardization evolves to an extreme the program would approximate the rigid rules option and would pose no new cost-estimating problems. Focusing, as we do here, on a program with certification by independent practitioners facilitates examination of the range of cost-estimating problems that a Medicare type C program might pose. Identifying where in this range a program would actually lodge, of course, presents an additional forecasting problem.

Estimating costs that would be imposed by such a program requires information on the behaviors of clients and families in seeking out care and information on the prescribing/certifying behaviors of physicians under the particular conditions established by the program—its benefit package, cost sharing, and so forth. The important point to stress is that under these program conditions, utilization cannot be forecast by application of rigid rules to data on the distribution of the population by prescription-relevant characteristics. Rules are not rigid; prescribers and users have room for maneuver that will make utilization depend, to a significant extent, on the particular incentives created by the program. This has implications for the process necessary to obtain information to assist in the cost-estimating task.

In discussing information needs and the potential for obtaining this information through experimental means, it is important to distinguish between the seeking behavior of potential recipients and the prescribing behavior of physicians or others authorized to prescribe services. The same information needs and problems that were discussed with reference to seeking behavior under rigid rules apply here and will not be discussed. However, unlike in the rigid rules policy, the prescriber would, at least initially, have great flexibility as to the types and quantities of services that are ordered. It, therefore, might be of great value to obtain information about likely prescribing behavior. Furthermore, we would argue that examination and evaluation of prescribing behavior is more amenable to the time and budget constraints imposed by social experimentation.

In anticipation of the potentially higher costs associated with a policy of this sort, it might make a certain amount of sense to begin to examine the feasibility of alternative cost containment strategies that might be required to make this policy a viable option. Attempts at cost control under this program could take one of two forms. Incentives for efficient behavior could be introduced, or prescribing behavior could be monitored or possibly regulated. Correspondingly, research with regard to estimated program costs for those that enter the system can also take two forms. For example, research can be conducted on the feasibility and cost consequences of capitating long-term-care clients. This approach would be consistent with the goal of developing incentives for efficient behavior. In contrast, a monitoring or regulatory approach would investigate the feasibility of establishing norms of practice with regard to prescribing long-term-care services. Although the problems of short-run versus long-run behavior may also be an issue here, we think that the magnitude of this potential problem is far smaller then with regard to seeking behavior. The extent of this problem would, to a large degree, be determined by how radically the delivery system and key decision makers were altered.

Conclusions

Although our conclusions derive primarily from analysis in this paper, they also are shaped by certain of our understandings about related matters. These are made explicit here. First, the economic and budgetary situation, for the foreseeable future, augurs ill for expensive new initiatives and favors policy changes whose costs can be forecast and whose cost-effectiveness can be established. Second, knowledge about which services work for which people is relatively weak, whether judged by effectiveness in retarding decline, maintaining living standards, or compensating for debility. Certainly, minimal levels of nutrition, heat, and other environmental matters can be identified; there is no excuse for not providing these. But much of the debate over long-term care concerns social and health services beyond this minimum; and we would argue that the effectiveness of these, individually and in combination, is not known. Third, although long-term-care benefits are not likely to be expanded greatly in the near term, substantial funding will flow into research on long-term-care issues over the next few years.

The discussion of this paper, together with these points, suggests the following conclusions:

1. If feasible, research should be conducted to identify the social, health, medical, and financial services that are most cost effective in retarding decline, maintaining standards of living, and compensating for debility for individuals with specified characteristics. Research focused on the retardation of decline should be clinically controlled and should not be incorporated in research that seeks simultaneously to identify demands or to explore the merits of various ways of organizing the provision of services. Although the research proposed here would be valuable, its feasibility may reasonably be questioned. For this reason, feasibility and planning studies should first be conducted. Long-term-care research attention and dollars are increasingly being directed at system-level research. Focused on organizational issues, this research is intended to reveal provision arrangements that will match services correctly with clients and that will induce efficient production; with the suggestion sometimes made that individual-level treatment efforts also will be identified. However, for reasons discussed above, treatment effects will only fortuitously be identifiable in the course of such research. Consequently, separate individual-level and system-level research is required. In sequence, individual-level research would seem the prior task, for the results of individual-level research, if obtainable, would be critically important both in designing provision arrangements and in judging the performance of provision alternatives.

The arguments favoring individual-level research in long-term care are reinforced by current fiscal pressures. In the absence of improved information about which services work, and how much, and for which kinds of people, it will be difficult to improve our effectiveness in assigning specific services (or resource amounts) to individuals; difficult to increase the cost effectiveness of long-term-care benefits; and virtually impossible to measure and describe the human benefits of long-term-care policy.

These implied benefits of individual-level research could be increased depending on the routinization of prescribing benefits. Feasibility studies and research focused on treatment effects would, therefore, yield a spin-off benefit. They would generate insights about the practicality of more routinized prescription and about limits to the reduction of discretion in the prescribing of service. Even in the absence of definitive conclusions about treatment effects, use of fixed prescribing rules might result in greater horizontal equity in the distribution of benefits.

2. Large-scale experiments should not be conducted to identify the service demands that would surface under various long-term-care policies that differ in organization, cost sharing, and other characteristics. A "Medicare part C" program, or other program that broadens benefits and open-endedly funds the individual service prescriptions of physicians or other independent professionals, would increase the quantity of service sought. Although supply constraints could determine utilization, great interest attaches to the utilization and costs of such programs were demands to be met. Would people increase utilization, substitute formal for informal care, and cause costs to skyrocket, or would demands be moderate and the program affordable? These are exceedingly important questions. However, we have argued above that they are probably inaccessible to feasible experimental research carried out over a period that is long by social experiment research standards (3–5 years). The high demands feared by some analysts would develop only as a real program was fully accepted and as families adjusted to a permanent change in their environment. These changes may be inhibited even in a well-conducted, very large social experiment. Consequently, our guess is that experimental findings of modest demands would be rejected as the basis for forecasts of demands under a real program.

The cost, infeasibility, and dubious outcome of experimentally based demand research in long-term care causes us to reject a research direction that we formerly might have favored. This implies rejection of open-ended policy options unless utilization control is assured, since in today's fiscal climate such options are unlikely to be accepted without knowledge of their cost implications. It also suggests that if benefits are broadened to include noninstitutional services, policy should be changed incrementally—not with respect to service coverage which could be broadened quickly and significantly, but with respect to the categories of persons offered new, noninstitutional services. Policy changes also should be structured to facilitate the collection of information that will aid in studying demand patterns.

3. From the perspective of the federal government, the expenditure

issues raised by mandating serious broadening of the Medicaid program are questions, to a significant degree, of state behaviors. These state behaviors, rather than individuals' needs and utilization, should be the subject of any research designed to illumine the expenditure implications of a broadening Medicaid benefit.

4. A block grant for long-term care does not pose a cost forecasting issue. However the block grant approach does pose questions about state behaviors with respect to the disposition of grant funds and the substantive implementation of policies. These merit serious research attention, if moves in the block grant direction are at all likely in long-term care.

5. A large-scale national survey should be conducted to identify the distribution of persons in and outside of institutions by functional and health status and by social and economic resources. This may be a relatively noncontentious note on which to conclude. The information produced by such a survey would be valuable in forecasting costs under virtually all program options and would be useful in studying a host of other issues.

Our broad conclusion is that the research required to support cost forecasting efforts is determined by the nature of the policy whose cost is to be forecast. Different policies will dictate radically different research. Consequently, some specification of policy possibilities and probabilities is key in designing a research strategy. More narrowly, we conclude that long-term-care research should be directed somewhat more at the individual level and, possibly, somewhat less at the system level. System-level research of the type now being planned can illumine organizational issues; but it cannot simultaneously tell us much about the merits of alternative treatments or about the outer bounds of demand for long-term-care services. Treatment effects are important. If they are shown to be accessible to feasible impact research at the individual level, such research should be conducted. Long-term-care demands also are very important. However, we have argued that information about them is likely to be inaccessible through feasible experimental research. Information about demands will more likely be obtained through research tied to policy changes that expand eligibility incrementally. Finally, policies incorporating substantial state control raise an additional set of forecasting issues. If such policies are seriously contemplated, different research focused on state behaviors is suggested.

Notes

1. For example: U.S. Congress, Congressional Budget Office, *Long-Term Care for the Elderly and Disabled,* Budget Issues Paper (Washington, D.C.: Government Printing Office,

1977); Federal Council on the Aging, *Report on National Policy for the Frail Elderly,* a working paper presented to the Federal Council, Washington, D.C.; U.S. Department of Health, Education, and Welfare, *Report of the Task Force on Long-Term Care/Community Services Reform;* Office of the Secretary, U.S. Department of Health, Education, and Welfare Internal Memorandum, Washington, D.C., July 14, 1978.

2. Because the incorporation of rigid rules so dominates a policy from our perspective, the description of this policy can neglect dimensions that are discussed in the other three caricatures. As a result, this caricature may appear more abstract than those that follow.

3. Fixed budgets are logically inconsistent with rigid rules policies. However, to argue, as does the text, that under a rigid rules policy federal funding "would have to be open-ended," one must overstate the hold that logical consistency has on the U.S. Congress. Thus, note that the rigid rules food stamp program is now funded with a fixed budget. It is not yet clear how Congress will adjust when the inconsistency of those two policy characteristics becomes apparent.

4. As will be argued in a later section of this paper, policy objectives should dictate the nature of the prescribing rules.

5. If "restrictive" ongoing policies are anticipated, then fears about "excessive" costs fueled by "excessive" demands may be misplaced. Furthermore, demands should not be the primary target of forecast-enabling utilization research. Instead, attention should focus on the response of service supplies to alternative financing and organizational policies. Interestingly, in examining the most expansive of their options, the Congress Budget Office anticipated demands that would consistently exceed supply. Consequently, their cost forecasts for that policy were entirely determined by estimates of the rate at which supplies would increase. See U.S. Congress, Congressional Budget Office, *Long-Term Care: Actuarial Cost Estimates* (Washington, D.C.: Government Printing Office, 1977).

6. For a more complete evaluation of past long-term-care demonstration projects, the readers is referred to J. Greenberg, D. Doth, A. Johnson, and C. Austin, *A Comparative Analysis of LTC Demonstration Projects: Lessons for Future Inquiry,* Project Share, forthcoming.

7. For example, see C. Austin and F. Seidl, "Validating Professional Judgment," *Health and Social Work,* forthcoming.

8. Although policy is rarely forged out of agreement on objectives, the clarification both of objectives and of their policy implications is important in developing policy options. For this reason, an analysis of long-term-care objectives would figure far more prominently and centrally in a paper focused on the design of policy than it does in this paper focused on research for policy.

9. If set in an income maintenance context, this objective would have different implications for the distribution of benefits. That option, however, fits more appropriately in the discussion of the second objective, maintenance of minimum standard of living.

10. J. P. Acton, *Measuring the Monetary Value of Lifesaving Programs* (Rand Corporation, 1970), p. 5675.

11. M. Derthick, *Uncontrollable Spending for Social Service Grants* (Brooking Institution, 1975).

12. David Doth, "Estimating the Impact of Expanded Medicaid Benefits for Community Based Long Term Care," Center for Health Services Research, University of Minnesota, April, 1980 (memorandum).

13. R. P. Nathan, et al., "Monitoring Block Grant Programs for Community Development," *Political Science Quarterly* 92, no. 2 (Summer 1977).

14. R. A. Hudson, *A Block Grant to the States for Long-Term Care,* Brandeis University, May 1977 (mimeo).

List of Contributors

James J. Callahan, Jr.
Director, Levinson Policy Institute and
Deputy Director, University Health Policy Consortium
Brandeis University
Waltham, Mass.

Lewis H. Butler
Adjunct Professor of Health Policy
University of California
San Francisco, Calif.

Paul W. Newacheck
Senior Research Associate
Health Policy Program
University of California
San Francisco, Calif.

Judith W. Meltzer
Research Associate
School of Social Service Administration
University of Chicago
Chicago, Ill.

William D. Fullerton
Principal, Health Policy Alternatives, Inc.
Silver Spring, Md.

Tom Joe
Research Associate, Senior Study Director
National Opinion Research Center
Center for the Study of Social Policy
Washington, D.C.

William Pollak
Associate Professor
School of Social Service Administration
University of Chicago
Chicago, Ill.

Harold A. Richman
Research Associate
Center for the Study of Social Policy
National Opinion Research Center
    and
Hermon Dunlap Smith Professor
University of Chicago, School of Social Service
    Administration
Chicago, Ill.

Elizabeth Ann Kutza
Associate Professor
School of Social Service Administration
University of Chicago
Chicago, Ill.

Robert L. Kane
Senior Researcher
Rand Corporation
Santa Monica, Calif.
    and
Professor, School of Medicine and School of Public Health
University of California at Los Angeles
Los Angeles, Calif.

Rosalie A. Kane
Social Scientist
Rand Corporation
Santa Monica, Calif.
    and
Lecturer, School of Social Welfare
University of California at Los Angeles
Los Angeles, Calif.

Jay Greenberg
Associate Director
Center for Health Services Research
    and
Assistant Professor
University of Minnesota
Minneapolis, Minn.

Frank Farrow
Senior Study Director
Center for the Study of Social Policy
National Opinion Research Center
Washington, D.C.

Index